CHAKRA
Healing for
DOGS

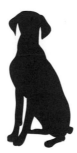

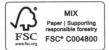

Published in 2022 by OH! Life
An imprint of Welbeck Non-Fiction Limited, part of Welbeck Publishing Group.
Based in London and Sydney.
www.welbeckpublishing.com

Text © Lynn McKenzie 2022
Design © Welbeck Non-Fiction Limited 2022
Illustrations by Sian Summerhayes © Welbeck Non-Fiction Limited 2022

Cover images: Sian Summerhayes © Welbeck Non-Fiction Limited (front);
Shutterstock/Anne Mathiasz and /majivecka (back), /Nadzeya Shanchuk (spine).

A CIP catalogue record for this book is available from the British Library.

ISBN 978-1-83861-101-9

Associate Publisher: Lisa Dyer
Copyeditor: Katie Hewett
Designer: Lucy Palmer
Production Controller: Felicity Awdry
Indexer: Angie Hipkin

Printed and bound in Dubai

10 9 8 7 6 5 4 3 2 1

CHAKRA
Healing for
DOGS

Energy work for a happy and healthy canine friend

LYNN MCKENZIE

Illustrations by Sian Summerhayes

CONTENTS

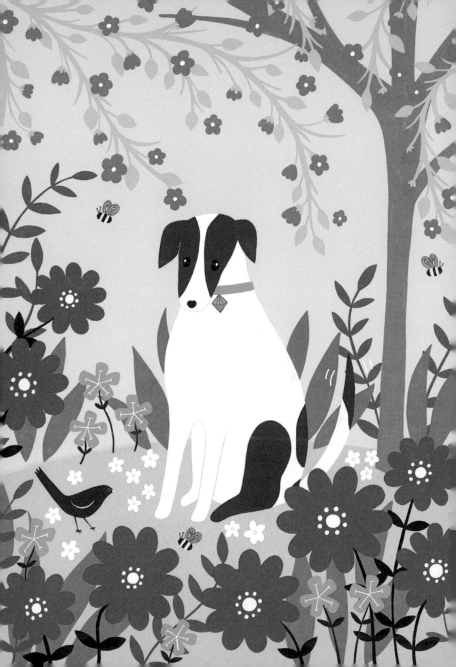

PREFACE

In 1993, my adorable light blonde English golden retriever pup, Jiggs, arrived in my life. I was thrilled to finally have him with me in the flesh and all I could think about was the fun, love and joy we had waiting for us. But as it often goes, God, the Universe or whatever you call your higher power had other ideas. Within a few short weeks, Jiggs became ill. We saw many vets, but Jiggs' constant and varied symptoms evaded conventional medicine.

After a great deal of anguish, I came to realize that it was my responsibility to get him well myself – and thus began my initiation into the world of healing dogs. I'd already been trained as a healer for humans, but this catapulted me into a complete change: career, lifestyle and location. Jiggs became the guide and teacher who entrenched me firmly on my new path, and I have never looked back.

I created *Chakra Healing for Dogs* to teach – and awaken you to – all that Jiggs taught me about healing and the chakras of dogs. You'll learn what they are; where they are located; how you can detect and balance them for greater health and wellbeing for your canine companion; how you can connect more closely with your dog; and even how your own chakras are connected to your dog's. Part One discusses the energy field and how it relates to balancing the chakras to heal and benefit your dog. In Part Two, you'll learn all about the major and minor chakras. Part Three details methods for whole-body energy work using crystals, flower essences and elixirs, colour therapy and Reiki.

Please also note that when we refer to your dog as "she", we are talking about both female and male dogs. Also, the terms "chakra balancing", "chakra clearing" and "chakra healing" are used interchangeably. Always err on the side of safety and consult a veterinarian to rule out illness if you observe any changes in your dog's health or behaviour. With all these things in mind, prepare to embark on a healing journey that may very well provide positive and memorable experiences for both you and your canine friend.

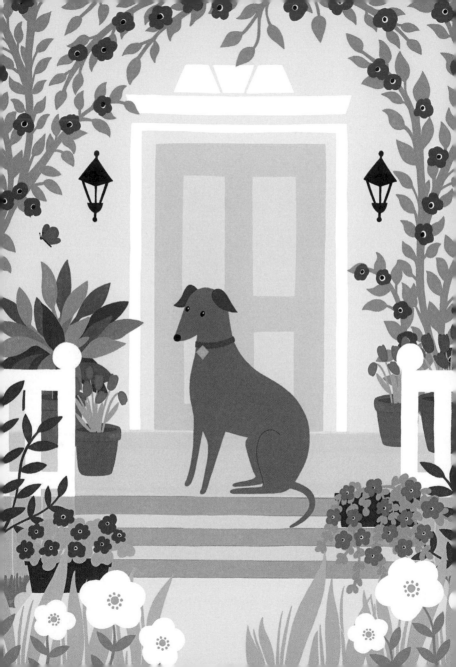

PART ONE
UNDERSTANDING YOUR DOG

Just as it does in humans, the chakra system holds the key to so many imbalances in our canine companions, whether they are of a physical, emotional or spiritual nature. By unlocking these imbalances, we not only enable our dogs to live in greater comfort and joy, but we can unravel their untold stories – sometimes even more effectively than through animal communication.

There are two approaches to use when balancing your dog's chakras. If your dog has a specific issue she needs help with, you can look up the corresponding chakra(s) and work with it or them. You can also use the energy methods described here to determine which of your dog's chakras need balancing and set the intention that working from this perspective will help alleviate any current or future issues. An additional benefit is that the healing journey is often mutual – so we can heal ourselves as we heal them. Thus, we work together towards knowledge, healing and growth while deepening our bonds with one another.

THE PSYCHIC CONNECTION

You are psychic – and you have a psychic connection with your dog! Did you know that? Perhaps without even thinking about it, you somehow know how your dog feels, what she wants or needs, and possibly even her innermost thoughts. This goes beyond just reading the normal body language of your canine friend or her subtle nuances to the deep connection the two of you share. You may not be fully conscious of it, but on some level, you just know; your spiritual lives are intertwined.

If some or all of this does not yet resonate with you just yet, don't let this concern you. It's something that will develop naturally and by osmosis – and with a little intention, focus and what you're about to learn from this book thrown in. I would bet that even if you are not aware of it, you've already begun to connect with your canine companion. Conversely, your dog also knows the true inner you: your deepest thoughts, feelings, needs and desires. And this goes beyond the invisible stuff like feelings and emotions, carrying through to the material plane and anything that is going on within your physical body. So how is that possible and how does this work?

Each of us (both ourselves and our canine friends) has an aura – a field of energy surrounding our physical bodies (which you'll learn about later). When we spend time with one another, our energy fields naturally intermingle and share space. It's in this place and time that we become familiar with and absorb energies from each other. This is the entry point into the way we "read" one another and our ailments, as well as exchanging information and even types of communication. Our dogs love to share space and energy with us, and if you happen to be a healer or are training to be one, you know how drawn your canine friend is to any form of energy healing or spiritual work.

If you don't yet have experience with healing, don't worry. Anyone can learn to heal dogs, and likewise, your dog can heal you too. This place of mutual healing begins with the basics of connecting and communicating with your canine companion. That shared space of your energy fields and the connection you already have with your dog is a great place to start – and the psychic link can open up a deeper level of communication that further strengthens your bond.

Tuning in to your dog on a deeper level will allow you to learn anything your dog might want you to know – they can be small things or bigger, more important things. It will give you a greater insight into your dog's overall wellbeing, including information related to the physical, emotional, mental and even spiritual aspects. Yes, your dog is a spiritual being!

There are a few methods through which we learn more about our dogs on a deeper level, and the more we practise, the easier it will become. Sometimes we may sense what our dog is experiencing; alternatively, we may learn by seeing, feeling, hearing or simply knowing. At other times, we may need to tune in deliberately and actively in order to determine our dog's wellbeing and current state or anything else your dog wants to communicate to you.

Communication through Imaging

If you try communicating with your canine friend and don't feel as if it is working straight away, don't give up. This skill can take time to develop, and it can depend on your openness, past training and current level of experience. However, one of the most important things you can do for success in connection and healing is to quieten your mind, especially any negative inner voices that may rear their ugly heads. Disruptive thoughts or distractions can muddy the psychic link and may prevent you from receiving communication clearly. Since our connections with our canine friends can often manifest in the form of images, if you feel stumped about what your dog is trying to tell you, it can help to imagine what that might be. Then go with whatever pops into your head first, as imagination is simply "imaging". This helps to prime the pump for a greater connection and further opening in communication.

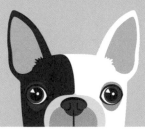

Connecting Energy Fields

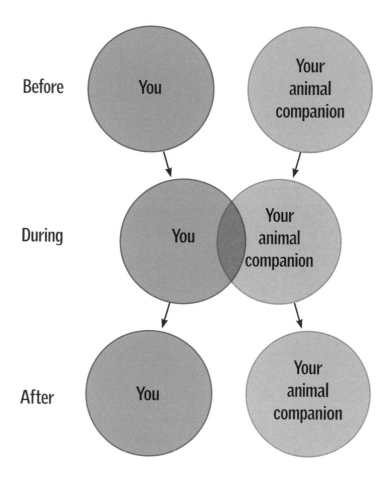

Before

During

After

Connecting Energies

1. Create a space as free from noise and distraction as possible where you can relax, undisturbed, and refer to the diagram on page 13.

2. To begin with, uncross your arms and legs, straighten your back, and bring yourself into a relaxed and comfortable position – either sitting or lying down.

3. Close your eyes if you are in a position to do so. Take a couple of deep breaths, inhaling through the nose and exhaling through the mouth. As you breathe in, visualize breathing in universal white light healing energy and exhaling any worries, fears or doubts you may have.

4. Now, visualize your energy field or aura as an orb around you that encompasses your physical body plus an extra 3–6 ft (1–2 m) around you.

5. Next, I'd like you to visualize your dog and visualize their energy field or aura as an orb around them. This orb encompasses their physical body plus an extra 1–2 ft (30–60 cm), depending on their size.

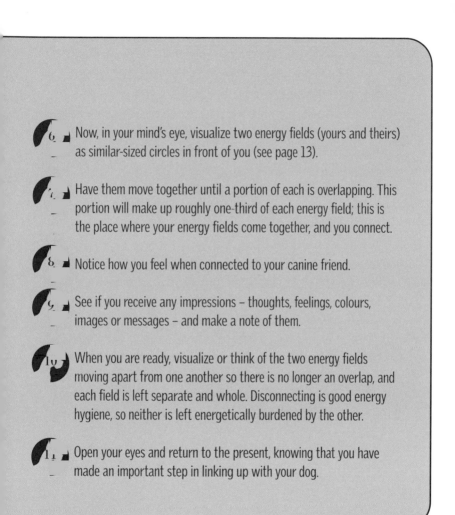

6 Now, in your mind's eye, visualize two energy fields (yours and theirs) as similar-sized circles in front of you (see page 13).

7 Have them move together until a portion of each is overlapping. This portion will make up roughly one-third of each energy field; this is the place where your energy fields come together, and you connect.

8 Notice how you feel when connected to your canine friend.

9 See if you receive any impressions – thoughts, feelings, colours, images or messages – and make a note of them.

10 When you are ready, visualize or think of the two energy fields moving apart from one another so there is no longer an overlap, and each field is left separate and whole. Disconnecting is good energy hygiene, so neither is left energetically burdened by the other.

11 Open your eyes and return to the present, knowing that you have made an important step in linking up with your dog.

Be open to receiving anything your dog might send your way and take notice of everything you pick up. Even if it feels unconventional, uncomfortable or unexpected – or if you think it may have come from you – don't discount it. Sometimes the most subtle of communications can seem like our own thoughts, but it's important to pay attention to everything you receive, even if it doesn't make sense straight away. You might even receive short "lightning" bursts of information, feelings, sensations or energy; these are especially important to take note of. Picture your mind as an empty canvas or a blank book, ready to receive, and then allow the page to fill with your dog's message. The more open you are to the connection, the more you will receive, and the more receptive you will be to assessing and healing your canine companion.

The gift of connecting psychically with our dogs is an innate one, and acknowledging the psychic link and trusting your own intuition are vital in the connection process. Your instinct is there for a reason, and it can help guide you through connecting and communicating with your dog. This often requires some level of letting go, especially of doubts, expectations and control. Attempts at connection may not go the way you might expect; allow the process to flow naturally. This will create and strengthen a psychic link that is clean and pure, providing a foundation for clearer, stronger connection and bonding. Trust your dog and your connection and follow it wherever it leads.

If you feel like anything is blocking your connection, take some time to visualize letting go of that blockage and shift your focus to the energy field connection you share with your dog.

Clearing a Blockage

To clear a blockage in your connection to your dog, try the following exercise.

 Visualize a physical representation of the blockage, then watch it turn to dust, fall to the ground and be swept away.

 Next, picture the connection between your heart and brow chakras to the heart chakra of your dog (see page 19) and allow your energy fields to mingle (see page 13).

 You can even visualize your energy fields coming together and overlapping, and then stay receptive to see what you sense or feel.

(We will cover energy fields more in depth in the next section, so don't worry if you feel like you need more information.)

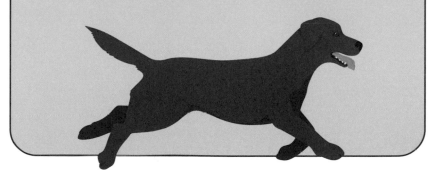

As humans, it can take some time to get used to opening the psychic link with our canine companions. Have patience with yourself and keep practising. Your dog is already open and is sharing with you and her canine friends naturally; it's second nature to her. But it is us who have to take the leap and stretch ourselves outside our comfort zones to awaken these innate gifts and abilities that allow us to receive the information. Once you establish the psychic connection with your dog from your perspective, it will always be there for you, and you will find it becomes easier to reconnect from there.

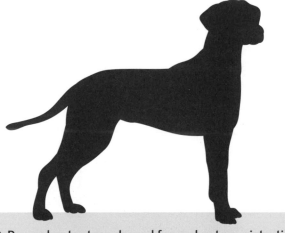

 TIP: Remember to stay calm and focused, set your intention, be open to whatever comes your way, and you'll undoubtedly feel a closer connection to your canine companion in no time.

Jiggs' Telepathic Pyramid

The image shows your connection (or psychic link) with your dog.

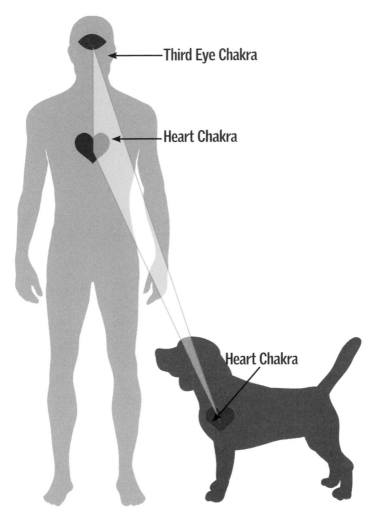

Third Eye Chakra

Heart Chakra

Heart Chakra

THE ENERGY FIELD

To learn about the chakras, first it is important to have a general understanding of the entire energy field – or energy body, as it's often called – and a knowledge of the way it works. The energy field is an invisible but vital component of any living being, and much like ours, our canine companion's energy field is comprised of three major components: the aura, the meridians and the chakras.

The Subtle Bodies or Aura

The aura is comprised of various layers of energy bodies, often called subtle bodies. Subtle bodies are layers of energy surrounding your canine companion's body, similar to a set of Russian dolls. The physical body makes up the innermost layer, followed by the etheric double, the emotional body and the spiritual body. The following is an image showing the aura and various layers of subtle bodies in a dog.

The Subtle Bodies

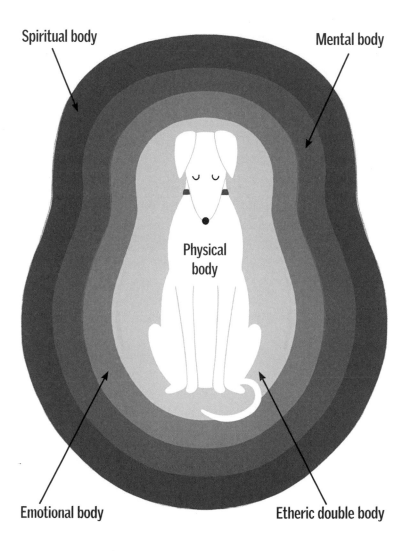

Spiritual body

Mental body

Physical body

Emotional body

Etheric double body

Meridians

Meridians, a concept in traditional Chinese Medicine that has moved into the mainstream in more recent times, are pathways through which life force energy flows. In very simplistic terms, you can think of meridians as etheric veins running throughout your dog's body, through which energy is transported. Studies have been carried out to prove that the vital organs and bodily systems rely on this energy as they rely on food, blood and air to survive.

Chakras

Chakras are energy vortexes, or portals, located in various spots throughout the body. Spinning and emanating outwards, chakras are vehicles for the assimilation of vital life force energy. This life force energy is filtered into a dog through their chakras and then through their entire being. When there are imbalances or blockages, these can inhibit assimilation, resulting in physical, emotional or behavioural symptoms. It's important to note that chakras are like cones, originating at points on the midline of the body, like stems, and fanning outwards through each of the layers of the subtle body.

To make things simple, if this concept is new to you, you can compare the subtle body, or aura, to the physical body; the chakras to the organs; and the meridians to the veins. This is a very basic approach, but it may help beginners to remember the different parts of the energy field.

Let's delve a little deeper into chakras. The word "chakra" is a Sanskrit word meaning "wheel", and the chakras are often referred to as "wheels of light" or "wheels of life". The concept originated in India over 4,000 years ago, and chakras are commonly referred to today in yoga and healing practices.

Chakras tell a story

Chakras can be regarded as "maps of consciousness" of an individual being, as they can tell the story of what has taken place in the experience and life of a dog – from surgeries to traumas and emotional upsets. The chakra system is where our canine companions receive energetic sustenance. All vital life force energy is filtered into an animal's energetic body through these portals, the chakras, and is then funnelled via the meridians into the endocrine system (which consists of various glands). This is how it ends up impacting our canine friends on a physical level. The degree to which their chakras are healthy, balanced and whole plays a large part in the way this life force energy reaches and enriches them.

There are numerous vortexes of energy within your dog that can be called chakras. However, it is the nine major and thirteen minor chakras, which correlate with various states of health, wellbeing and consciousness, that we are going to concern ourselves with. Chakras can be seen or felt (by some) as spinning wheels of energy and resemble cones, with both a front and a back side, spinning in opposite directions. Think of the way you squeeze out a wet towel, with one hand twisting one way and the other hand twisting the other; this is similar to the way chakras flow.

The Chakra Vortex

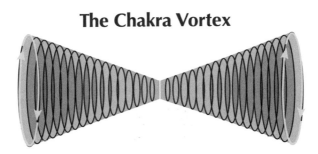

How Energy Flows to Our Dogs

Life Force Energy

Subtle Bodies

Negative thoughts and emotions can link with the normal life-force flow of energy and be carried into the physical.

Negative mental and emotional energy patterns passing through the subtle bodies or aura will interfere with the normal flow of energy into the physical level.

Chakra Portals

This in turn weakens the flow of energy into the chakras and their corresponding areas of the physical body.

Meridians

Nervous, endocrine and circulatory systems

Cells, tissues and organs of the physical body

This results in an imbalance and a buildup of negative energy, which is transmitted to the physical body and can manifest as illness or disease.

Chakra anatomy

Chakras vary in brightness, depth and size, and also in the amount of energy, from strong to weak, depending upon the health and vitality of your canine friend. Each chakra governs different glands and organs in the physical body, and each also relates to specific emotional, mental and spiritual aspects of consciousness. An animal's thoughts and feelings also filter through the chakras, eventually resulting in manifestations that show up in the physical body.

When energy does not flow freely in the chakras, your dog's body is not able to function properly. Stress of any kind – whether of a physical, emotional, mental or spiritual nature – can cause an imbalance in our animal companion's chakras. This imbalance can eventually lead to disease if it is not cleared and balanced by us.

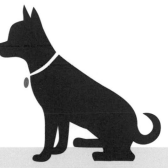

 TIP: It is important to remember that a situation or event that stresses one individual may not stress another, as some beings are much more sensitive than others.

Healing

We can alter the chakras through healing. It is also possible for other influences to alter them (in both positive and negative ways). It does not require any special talents for you to learn to heal your canine companions through their chakras – just a strong desire to do so and the intention to understand and help them. For some of you, simply using the chakra charts included in this book and placing your hands in the area of each chakra will be enough. You can also feel for the energy vortex or energy spin, and as you become accustomed to the feel of the chakras – and particularly your dog's chakras, as each dog is different – you may start to feel or sense whether they are balanced or not.

Locating the chakras

Please note that not all people will be able to see or feel their dog's chakras (see annotated images on pages 50–1 and 88–9). Over time, and with practice, most of us will be able to locate them in one way or another. If you're having difficulty, don't be discouraged; just maintain your trust and focus on what you intend to do, and use the chart provided as a guide. Either way, you can still perform beneficial healing and clearing work for your dog from wherever you are currently.

Ways to Find
the Chakras

Seeing: Actually seeing energy moving
or colour present in a chakra.

🐾

Feeling: Feeling definitive movement of
energy in the area of a chakra.

🐾

Sensing: Using your inner knowing and
guidance to determine where a chakra is located.

🐾

Dowsing: Using pendulum dowsing (if you know how)
to detect where a chakra is.

🐾

Kinesiology: Using muscle testing (if you know how)
to detect the location of a chakra.

We'll talk more about this and how to balance your dog's
chakras in Part Two.

WORKING WITH DOGS

Whether your dog is a puppy, an elderly dog or mature adult in her prime, we approach chakra (and other) healing work the same way for each individual. Unfortunately, in today's world, there are many dogs who have been subject to abuse, trauma, abandonment, the rescue system and more, as well as stray dogs (which thankfully are rare in many regions but unfortunately are more abundant in others) who have had little to no interaction with humans and who are mostly undomesticated. Most of you will probably be applying the practices you learn in this book to help your own domesticated dogs, but you can also take the skills you learn here and help to heal any dog, including rescued, abused, traumatized, abandoned, lost and even stray dogs; either those still living in the wild or those who have been rehomed so they can live a happier and more comfortable life. Dogs and puppies who have been rescued, abused, traumatized, abandoned or are strays require special concessions when it comes to healing.

Signs Your Dog Is Unwell

Always contact your veterinarian if you notice any changes in your dog, whether physical or behavioural. Watch for alterations in her eating, drinking, digestion and elimination habits as well as notable mood or other normal routine changes. Issues such as excessive hunger, refusing to eat, vomiting, diarrhoea, constipation, hair loss, sudden bad breath, eye or nose discharge, pupil dilation, wounds or swelling, lethargy or hiding from you should always be considered signs of potential illness until otherwise ruled out.

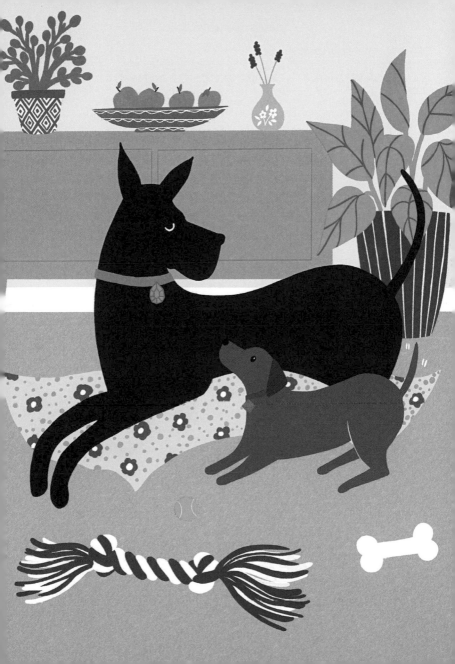

Taking Stock and Degrees of Sensitivity

Before beginning any healing work on your dog, always take stock of how delicate an otherwise healthy dog or puppy might be – physically, emotionally and mentally – as this will vary from being to being. Think of dogs as falling into categories of low, medium and high sensitivity.

Low sensitivity: A large proportion of dogs fall into this category, particularly those who live with families and are used to noise and regular handling.

Medium sensitivity: I consider a puppy , elderly dog or a dog who has just had surgery to be much more delicate than average, so I'd place them in this group.

High sensitivity: I would place abused, traumatized, abandoned, rescued and stray dogs in this group as they are often profoundly frightened, shocked and sometimes even terrified.

These are generalizations, of course, and as with all generalizations, there are exceptions to the rule. For the new healer, having these three categories is a good place to start, and as dogs are living beings, we would rather have you err on the side of caution of a dog having more sensitivity rather than less.

In general, dogs are one of the less sensitive of the domesticated species when it comes to energy and healing work, but there are exceptions to every rule, so it's very important consider them individually when working with them. One of the first rules of healing is to do no harm, and this includes never allowing your healing work to create additional stress in a dog. It is intended only to alleviate stress and tension and bring forth greater wellbeing.

Hands-on or Distance Healing

While most dogs may enjoy a hands-on approach to chakra healing and balancing, other, more sensitive, dogs will much prefer a hands-off method. This can be related to their specific sensitivity grouping mentioned opposite, with more delicate dogs being inclined to prefer distance work (but it's not always that way). Whether you're working hands-on or hands-off, your results should not vary. Performing hands-off or distance healing on your dog simply means conducting the healing method anywhere from a few feet to a continent away. This approach is just as effective and provides the same great results you'd get by working hands-on.

Preparing Your Dog for Chakra Work

Everything in this Universe is energy, and our canine friends are impacted by all of it – much more than you might expect. Dogs act as sponges for us, helping clear our energy, and they are also susceptible to their own imbalances. Aside from their own issues, the thoughts, feelings, mindsets and illnesses of those around them, planetary energies, injustices to their species as a whole, and even global energies like pandemics and wars impact them and can create imbalances. Because of this, healing is very beneficial for your dog, as it helps her to release all this unwanted, non-beneficial energy. The first step I recommend when preparing to work with your dog is to ground and protect her.

Please note, the following exercise can be done physically on the body, in the aura (about 4–6 in/10–15 cm above her body), or over distance – from across a room or even in another location. Always honour what your canine companion prefers. Sensitive animals generally prefer it to be performed off the body. If your canine friend has touchy paws, you can do the exercise hands-on, but then hold your hands above the paws when you get to that area. Our main goal is healing, so we don't want to add any extra stress.

If you are familiar with energy fields, as you're performing this exercise, visualize and set the intention that your dog's chakras, subtle bodies and meridians will come into perfect balance each time you do it.

As with ours, the energy field of animals can become imbalanced through stressors, the environment, shock, trauma and absorbing energy from others. This simple grounding exercise is designed to reconnect them with the energy of Mother Earth, which is the most natural state for any living being.

Grounding Your Dog's Energy

This exercise consists of a series of three strokes.

 To begin, bring yourself into a calm, focused state; take a few deep, cleansing breaths, releasing any stresses of the day.

 With the middle and index finger of each hand together (with the sides of each index finger touching), trace a line from the tip of your dog's nose up the middle of her face, between the eyes and ears, along the midline of the body (spine) to the shoulders, then separate your hands and bring one hand down each shoulder and leg to the top of her front paws. As you're doing this, visualize your dog's energy flowing along with it. At the paws, rest gently and visualize her energy going down through the floor and into the ground below, connecting deep with Mother Earth and releasing any non-beneficial energy. Let your dog or your intuition tell you how long to hold – generally between 30 seconds and two minutes – until you feel her energy connecting deep within the Earth.

 Repeat that stroke, but this time, go all the way to her hips before separating your hands and tracing down each back leg, as you did with the front legs in the first stroke. Again, visualize your dog's energy flowing along with the stroke and her energy going into the ground below, connecting deeply with Mother Earth. Hold for a time as before.

 Finally, repeat this once more, but go all the way to the tail and trace along to the tail tip (or what would have been the tail tip in an animal with a docked tail) and cup your hands there and hold, allowing for her energy to go down into the ground and connect her deeply with Mother Earth.

 When you have finished, visualize your dog's aura in a protective bubble of pink light (pink is for healing). The bubble should be permeable to loving energies and repel non-beneficial energies. To help this transpire, visualize hearts (as loving energies) coming towards the protective bubble of pink light surrounding your dog and permeating the bubble. Then visualize arrows (as non-beneficial energies) coming towards the protective bubble of pink light surrounding your dog and being repelled by the bubble.

HEALING PRINCIPLES

The principles of healing are underpinned by beliefs, intentions and wishes – our own and those of our companions – and our commitment to our work.

Our Beliefs

We believe that canines are sacred beings, just like all other beings, and that they have divine wisdom to share with us. We feel that they are in our lives for connection and healing as well as teaching and guidance.

We understand that through connection and communication, our dogs can help heal us and we can heal them. By building strong relationships with our dogs that transcend the physical plane, we are awakened to the deep connection we share. We recognize that canines help us navigate the circle of life and guide us throughout our existence in many ways.

Our dogs possess multiple levels of consciousness – physical, emotional, mental and spiritual – that allow us access for connection, communication and healing. We respect the sacredness of each of our dogs and listen intuitively to their responses, proceeding with the utmost care and respect.

We also respect our dog's wishes for healing and honour her preference for hands-on or distance techniques as desired. We release any judgements about the connection, communication, and healing of our canine friend and trust that her higher self, and our open heart, will lead us to a place of true healing for both of us.

Our Commitment

We commit to partnering with our canine friends and asking permission before beginning any connection or healing work. We draw upon our connection with our dog and work towards healing with an open mind, allowing her to guide her own journey for the highest good of all involved. We also commit to deferring to the expertise of a veterinary professional when necessary to diagnose any condition or ailment.

We commit to practising and fostering our own spiritual growth and self-healing in order to be a clear and strong channel for harmonious connection and restorative energy healing with our dogs. We trust our own hearts and wisdom and try our best to avoid allowing emotions to cloud our judgements or diminish our connection.

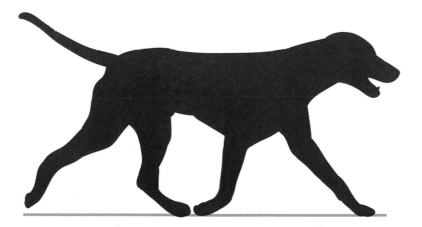

HEALING MODALITIES

The way we prepare ourselves to perform our healing work is just as important as the healing techniques themselves.

Ourselves as Conduits

When it comes to healing, it is important to recognize we are simply the conduits for the healing to take place; we are not the ones causing it. It is God, the Universe, or whatever higher power you subscribe to that creates and determines the final healing result. We always do our very best with the highest intention to help any living being, but if a being doesn't heal the way we envisioned, it's beyond our control and not our fault. I always ask that the healing be in accordance with divine order and for the "highest and best good" of the dog and all concerned, as there may be prior spiritual agreements or contracts at play. This never stops us from trying, though, as even in the death and dying process, healing work can be beneficial to your dog and healing can be received.

Preparing Ourselves for Chakra Work

When performing healing work, it's important to place ourselves into what is known as a "healing state". It's a peaceful state, similar to a meditative state, but where we're a little more alert and aware. Being in this state is as important (or even more so) than the accuracy of the healing techniques we perform.

Preparing for Healing Work

For best results:

Relax

🐾

Intensify your focus

🐾

Quiet any distracting mind chatter

🐾

Enter a peaceful, grounded and centred state

🐾

Adopt an unobtrusive energy resonance that creates an opening and space
for the dog to come to you (physically or energetically)

🐾

Set aside your ego mind

🐾

Move into your heart centre

🐾

Be highly respectful and non-judgemental

🐾

Ask the permission of the dog being you are about to work with

Setting Your Intention

Another important component is your intention; it's as important as the technique you employ when it comes to healing your furry friend. When you work on your dog's chakras, I recommend creating an intention for the end result of the healing work you do. Here are a couple of examples of what I mean:

"I intend that Juniper's inflammation and pain be eliminated."

"I intend to help Finn adapt to the houseguests we'll be having next week."

"I intend that Emma's spay surgery takes place smoothly and without incident."

"I intend that Camy's transition to the spirit realm happens smoothly and peacefully."

You can ask for anything when it comes to healing, whether it's a physical, emotional, mental or spiritual result; no goal or dream is too big. Even if your dog has an incurable or life-threatening disease, it doesn't hurt to ask for healing, as I've seen many miracles in my 30-plus years of doing this work. At the end of my intention, I always like to say, "I ask for this or something better, so be it."

Visualization

Visualization is another powerful healing tool. You can visualize the chakras, visualize which ones require balancing and visualize them coming into perfect balance. You will also use visualization in some of the other balancing tools.

Your Healing Team

Each of us has a team of benevolent beings that are willing and want to help us in our healing work. Mostly, they are beings who have already crossed over: ancestors, elders, loved ones – both human and animal – and even well-known beings like the patron saint of animals, St Francis of Assisi, or the clairvoyant Edgar Cayce. You don't have to know your healing team intimately, but I urge you to call them in to be with you when working on your dog.

Hands-on Healing

As the name implies, hands-on healing is done by placing your hands on or immediately above the body, in this case the chakra, and intending that universal healing energy flows to the animal and corrects any imbalance.

Distance Healing

Distance healing can be done anywhere, from a few feet to a continent away from the animal, while intending that universal healing energy flows to the animal and corrects any imbalance.

If you currently share your life with a canine friend, the chances are that you know her well enough to know whether she would prefer a hands-on or hands-off approach – but if not, just try each method and let her enthusiasm for and reaction to each tell you which one she prefers. A hands-on approach is preferred by many canines.

Sensing Your Dog's Chakras

 Once you're in a healing state, use the diagram on pages 50–1 to locate each of the chakras on your dog's body.

 Then, using your fingertips, start about 4–6 in (10–15 cm) above the body in the general area of each chakra, and slowly lower your fingers towards your dog's body at the chakra point. You can work in their energy field or directly on the body (more on this below). Determine, one by one, if you see (with your physical eyes or in your mind's eye), hear, feel or sense anything; some of you will and some of you won't, and all are equally fine.

If working hands-on, it's okay to hold your hand directly on your dog's body and continue feeling and sensing, as long as she is not in any way irritated or agitated by it. Some highly sensitive dogs will find this to be too much pressure, energetically speaking, even if you're barely touching her – so be sure to honour this. Some people will feel the chakra energy as a buzzing or tingling, as heat or cold or another sensation, even if it's very subtle – while others may have to work at it and practise over time to sensitize themselves to this subtle energy.

Determining Which of Your Dog's Chakras Is Out of Balance

Using the exercise opposite, you may be able to feel a subtle difference in your dog's chakras. Some chakras will feel like they are in perfect balance, while others may feel out of balance. Again, this may take some time and practise to determine. If you happen to know how to do muscle testing or dowsing, you can use either of these methods to determine or confirm which of your dog's chakras need balancing. You can also simply ask to be shown or told which chakras most need healing. The latter requires trust in your psychic/intuitive abilities.

If none of these options seems feasible to you, you can simply use the information provided in Part Two of this book to work on the chakra most relevant to your dog's symptoms, behaviours or conditions, or you can work on each of them in turn.

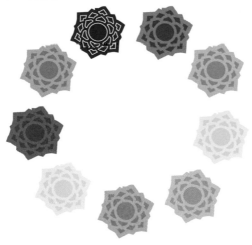

Balancing the Chakras

You can bring your dog's chakras into balance, one by one, by simply using a strong intention to do so while holding your hand over each chakra you are intending to balance. Then wait until it happens and until you feel it is complete. Becoming proficient at this requires lots of trust and a big leap of faith.

Another way to do this, and the one I use most frequently, is simply by using the healing statement I've included for each chakra. Here's an example:

> "I send red light to [dog's name]'s root chakra and ask that it come into perfect balance, spinning in an appropriate fashion, with any imbalances, blockages or non-beneficial energies being released to the spiritual. And so it is."

In this example, I used the colour (red) that is associated with the chakra I was balancing (the root chakra). To use this process for the chakras you intend to balance for your dog, see the information listed for each chakra in Part Two. You can also work with your dog's chakras using other methods, including:

Spirit animal
This is a more shamanic approach; each chakra has a related spirit animal. You can call in the spirit of the corresponding animal to come to your canine friend to heal, balance and clear her chakras and any and all related conditions.

Physical stimulation
Weak chakras can be stimulated physically with various activities, such as exercise, swimming, bathing or massage, depending on the particular chakra you are working on.

Archangels

Call in the archangel related to each chakra to come to your dog and assist with balance and clearing her chakras and any and all related conditions.

Affirmations

Use the affirmations provided for each chakra as they apply to your dog (be sure to customize them).

Visualization

Visualize the chakra in its current state, and then the way you'd like it to be. Then, on the count of three, visualize it coming into perfect balance. Then set the intention that it will "lock in" to this balanced fashion and remain balanced.

Pendulum Dowsing or Muscle Testing

If you know how to pendulum dowse or muscle test to determine which chakras most need balancing, you can employ these methods (see also page 54).

Brain Integration

This method balances the right and left hemispheres of the brain. Trace a figure of eight over the area of the chakra you want to balance for your dog, in her aura, with the intention of harmonizing the energy and bringing it into perfect balance (see also page 55). Visualize a number "8" on its side, like an infinity symbol but with more rounded loops; then, with the palm of your hand, trace the "8" from the centre down to the left and up and across the middle, then down to the right and up and across the middle. Trace 3–5 times, in the direction of the chakra you wish to balance, and then in the direction of the entire energy field.

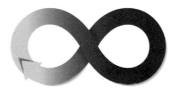

Sending Frequencies

Radionics, as it is known, is a technique that is conducted to send particularly restorative energetic frequencies to your dog for the purposes of promoting healing, and in this case, healing of a specific chakra. This can be done with a radionics machine or through your own intention and energy. If this topic interests you, I suggest further study. But for the sake of simplicity here, use the Sending Frequencies exercise below.

 Once you are in your healing state, you can send frequencies to your dog using the following statement along with a strong intention:

> **"I send [substance] to [dog's name] and ask that she receive it perfectly now, on all levels, all dimensions, all aspects, known and unknown, now and for all time."**

 Then visualize and intend that it is being received by your dog for as long as it is in her highest and best good. You can use this method to send crystals, colours or flower essences/gem elixirs, etc. to your dog.

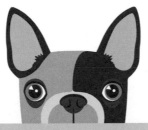

Examples of Sending Frequencies

"I send smoky quartz to Daisy and ask that she receive it perfectly now, on all levels, all dimensions, as aspects, known and unknown, now and for all time."

"I send the colour turquoise to River and ask that she receive it perfectly now, on all levels, all dimensions, as aspects, known and unknown, now and for all time."

"I send Bach Rescue Remedy to Wynter and ask that she receive it perfectly now, on all levels, all dimensions, as aspects, known and unknown, now and for all time."

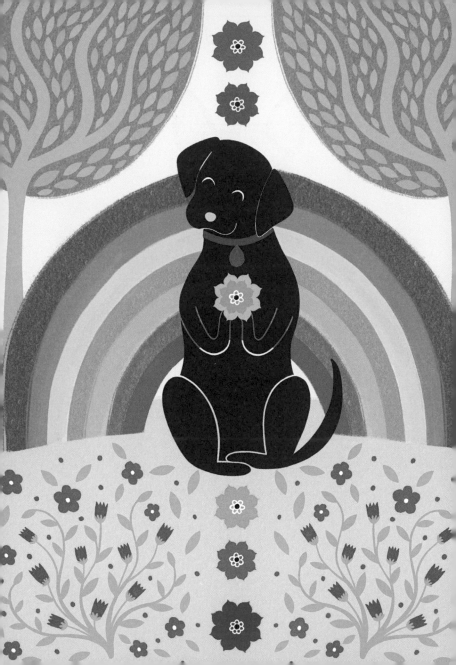

PART TWO
THE CHAKRAS

Each of your dog's chakras governs and relates to key qualities, areas, matters, issues, bodily systems, organs and emotions. Dogs have both major and minor chakras, with some of the major chakras being stand-alone chakras and others having associated minor chakras. For example, in the case of one of the major chakras, the root chakra, there are a number of related minor or sub-chakras that are associated with it and relate specifically to certain detailed components of it. The minor chakras associated with the root chakra are the following: the self-preservation, reproductive and digestive chakras. We will explore the major chakras first and then delve into the minor chakras.

THE MAJOR CHAKRAS

The health, wellbeing and balance of any chakra – major or minor – is impacted by life experiences. These can include anything and everything that occurs from the time of conception and birth, right through to the present moment in the lives of each dog, and it can also include past life issues. Because of this, puppies and dogs who have been through accidents, traumas, illnesses, surgeries, abuse, homelessness, puppy farms, etc. will almost always require more chakra clearing.

Generally speaking, when any being is exposed to stress, trauma, grief, etc., the imbalance that occurs in their energy field (and thus their chakra system) gravitates to their weakest area. In dogs, this is often the hind region – hence the more frequent occurrences of hip dysplasia and arthritis in dogs as compared to cats and other species. When you look at the chakras in the area of the hip (which you'll learn about later), you'll notice the root, the respect recognition and the self-preservation chakras are all in that area, and it's no coincidence that many of the more emotional and psychological issues in dogs, such as anxiety, aggression, distrust, fear, hyperactivity and timidity, are all related to these chakras.

Another example is that most domesticated dogs have either been spayed or neutered very young for population control, whether the timing is in their best interests or not. Therefore, the larger breeds especially can experience issues related to these surgeries being performed too early in life, which can impact their sexual progression chakra. This causes related concerns such as bone growth issues, incontinence and torn ACLs (anterior cruciate ligaments) in the knee.

A dog can have a chakra that's out of balance, with only one of the associated traits listed in the sections that follow being obvious to you, and sometimes even without any of the associated traits apparently present. Remember, matters of a physical, emotional, mental or spiritual nature can all impact a chakra – but not all are required for an imbalance to be present. Energy is a complex and vast topic, and the way it works and impacts our canine companions is not always linear. Be sure to trust your findings and balance her chakras whether you understand why they are out of balance or not.

Issues in our canines can impact more than one chakra, and healing them often crosses over to a number of chakras. Thus, don't be surprised if more than one is out of balance for your dog as a result of one issue or area of concern.

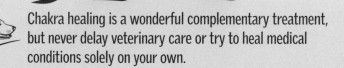

Chakra healing is a wonderful complementary treatment, but never delay veterinary care or try to heal medical conditions solely on your own.

The Nine Major Chakra Points

Like us, your dog's body is not just physical: it's made up of energy and the chakras are the major energy centres, or vortexes, that aid in the absorption and distribution of that energy.

Working with your dog's chakras to get them balanced, flowing and in harmony can keep her at peak health and wellness and allow her to recover from any physical or emotional trauma. Unlike us, dogs have an extra major chakra, the brachial (see pages 84–7).

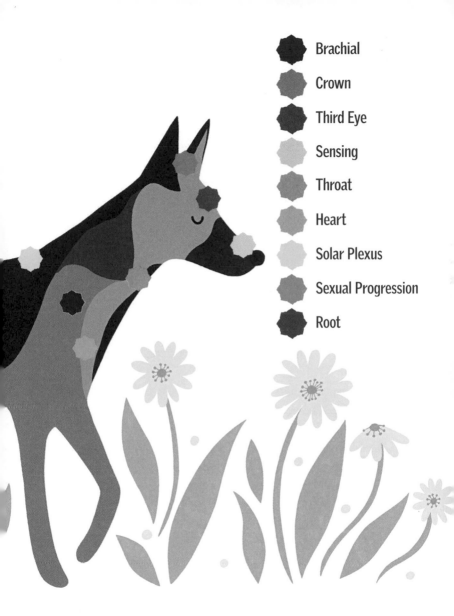

Brachial

Crown

Third Eye

Sensing

Throat

Heart

Solar Plexus

Sexual Progression

Root

Root Chakra
(Base Chakra)

The root chakra is related to issues of the physical world, health, strength, stability, nourishment, boundaries, self-preservation, survival instinct, feeling comfortable in their skin, feeling grounded and status in a family or pack (this includes the human and animal family – of both dogs and other species). Generational and early life wounds are found in this chakra, as well as energies related to the species as a whole. Connected to matters of safety, courage individuality, security, patience and instincts such as the fight-or-flight response.

Location: The root chakra is located at the coccyx, or base of the tail.

Associated colours: Red, coral red or sometimes black.

Associated glands/organs: Adrenals, kidneys, spine, colon, anus, hips, legs and paws, bones, blood.

Possible imbalance: Insecurity, fear, lack of trust, anxiety, arthritis, incontinence, dominance, territorial aggression, fear, aggression, resource guarding, blood issues and disorders, autoimmune disease, orthopaedic issues and disorders including bone growth issues, kidney disease, hip dysplasia, constipation, diarrhoea, anal gland issues, IBS or IBD.

🐾 A balanced root chakra can result in a dog who is in good health, vital, comfortable in her body, has a sense of trust in her world, feels safe and secure, has the ability to relax and be still, is stable, flourishing, generous and enjoys her role.

 An imbalanced root chakra can result in a dog who is fearful, distrusting, anxious or aggressive, fails to thrive, is timid, hyperactive, jealous and fearful of missing out, eats faeces, displays separation anxiety.

Spirit animal: The spirit or totem animal associated with the root chakra is the horse. The horse relates to courage, strength and stability. Call in or ask horse energy to come forth to your canine companion to be with her for the purpose of healing her root chakra.

Ways to stimulate the root chakra: Conduct a grounding exercise for your dog (see pages 32–3), give your dog a full-body massage or touch her gently all over to help her to connect better with her various body parts. Encourage exercise and spending time outdoors with her paws on the ground.

Archangel: Uriel is the archangel associated with the root chakra. You can call upon Archangel Uriel to ground your dog's energy through the root chakra and at the same time to release any and all non-beneficial energies to be transmuted by the spiritual realm. Feel free to list any specifics you are aware of as you ask for assistance from the archangels.

Affirmations: You can create your own affirmation to suit your dog's particular situation or use one of the following:
"[Dog's name] is happy, healthy and whole."
"[Dog's name] feels fully supported and loved."
"[Dog's name] trusts herself and her surroundings."

Visualization: If you've determined that the root chakra is imbalanced, first visualize it as it currently is, and then, on the count of three, visualize it coming into perfect balance. Then visualize "locking it in" to this balanced fashion so that it will stay balanced.

Crystal healing: There are a number of ways to work with crystals to help balance your dog's chakras. You can send the energetic frequency of a crystal to your dog; use a crystal physically on the body via a crystal massage, aura massage or simple touch; or place the crystal in an area your dog spends a lot of time, like under a dog bed or a chair cushion.

Pendulum dowsing: If you have already determined that your dog's root chakra is imbalanced, you can take a pendulum, and while holding it over the root chakra, physically spin it to the right while at the same time asking that her chakra comes into perfect balance "with any imbalances, blockages or non-beneficial energies to be released to the spiritual", as you say in the healing statement. Give it some time to begin to resonate with the swing of the pendulum. Then after minute or two, you can stop and use whatever method you used previously to recheck the root chakra.

Brain integration: Brain integration balances the right and left hemispheres of the brain. Trace figures of eight over the area of the root chakra, in the aura of your dog with the intention of harmonizing the energy and bringing it into perfect balance. Visualize a number "8" on its side, and then with the palm of your hand, trace the sideways "8", beginning in the centre, at the "X" (or where it crosses over). From the centre, come down to the left and up and around and across the middle, then down to the right and up and around and across the middle. Trace this pattern 3–5 times, first in the direction of the root chakra and then in the direction of the entire energy field.

CRYSTALS THAT AID IN HEALING THE ROOT CHAKRA

Black tourmaline

Boji stone

Garnet

Hematite

Jet

Red jasper

Ruby

Smoky quartz

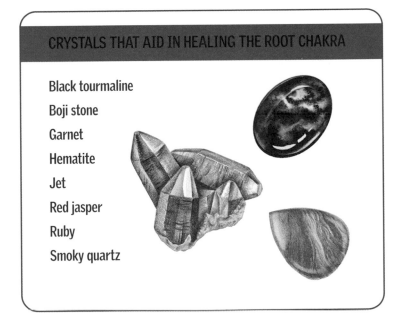

Sexual Progression Chakra (Sacral Chakra)

Related to all aspects of procreation and sexuality, including irregular heat cycles, natural mating instinct, drive to propagate the species, marking territory, hormone imbalances, false pregnancies, mammary gland issues, inbreeding deficiencies, inherited disorders, spay and neuter issues and time spent in puppy farms. Also affects sense of purpose, empowerment, mood, nurturing, assimilation of food, imbalanced emotions, lack of confidence, low energy, vitality and creativity.

Location: Lower abdomen to navel area.

Associated colour: Orange.

Associated glands/organs: Spleen, intestines, bladder, the internal and external male and female reproductive organs including ovaries, testicles, prostate and uterus.

Possible imbalance: Any breeding issues including infertility, spay and neuter issues, and hormone imbalances (irregular heat cycles). Lack of confidence, skittishness, easily startled, hyperactive, weak, high stress or aggression regarding crate and/or car rides, cystitis, urinary tract issues, incontinence, crystals, stones and blockages, low energy, lower back pain, asthma, allergies and coughs.

🐾 A balanced sexual progression chakra can result in a dog who is happy, joyful, confident, empowered and relaxed, well-nourished, energized, with no issues related the reproductive organs including spay or neuter surgeries, heat cycles or planned ethical breeding practices.

🐾 An imbalanced sexual progression chakra can result in a dog who has digestive issues, is malnourished, has difficulty conceiving, experiences deficiencies from inbreeding, marks territory, is highly emotional and moody, feels unsettled at home or exhibits signs of abuse suffered as a result of mistreatment or time spent in a puppy mill. Also difficulties arising from spay/neuter surgery.

Spirit animal: The spirit or totem animal associated with the sexual progression chakra is the spider. The spider relates to creativity, intuition, feminine energy and the weaving of fate. Call in or ask spider energy to come forth to your canine companion to be with her for the purpose of healing her sexual progression chakra.

Ways to stimulate the sexual progression chakra: Massage (hands on the body or massage the energy field in the aura), bathing and swimming are great options.

Archangel: Chamuel is the archangel associated with the sexual progression chakra. You can call upon Archangel Chamuel to balance your dog's energy related to the sexual progression chakra, and at the same time to release any and all non-beneficial energies to be transmuted by the spiritual realm. Feel free to list any specifics you are aware of as you ask for assistance from the archangels.

Affirmations: You can create your own affirmation to suit your dog's particular situation or use one of the following:
"[Dog's name] is at one with spay/neuter policies."
"[Dog's name] is in touch with and processes her feelings."
"[Dog's name] is well-nourished."

Visualization: If you've determined that the sexual progression chakra is imbalanced, first visualize it as it currently is, and then, on the count of three, visualize it coming into perfect balance. Then visualize "locking it in" to this balanced fashion so that it will stay balanced.

For crystal healing, pendulum dowsing and brain integration: Refer to these sections under the root chakra section (see pages 54–5).

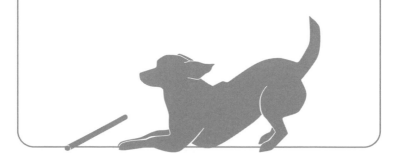

CRYSTALS THAT AID IN HEALING THE SEXUAL PROGRESSION CHAKRA

Brown jasper

Carnelian

Copper citrine

Fire agate

Moonstone

Orange calcite

Orange jade

Red coral

Red quartz

Salmon

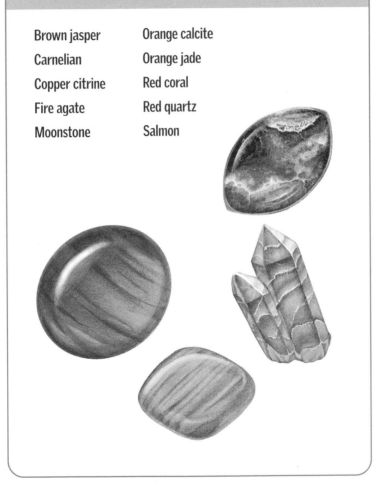

Solar Plexus Chakra

Related to issues of self-confidence, personal power and will. It affects the energetic centre of identity and personality of the dog and is considered to be one of the key centres for animals and humans to communicate physically, so it is therefore associated with how connected or disconnected a canine is to humans as well as other canines. It is also related to predator/prey issues in dogs. This chakra governs the sympathetic nervous system, digestive system, metabolism and emotions.

Location: Back mid-spine.

Associated colours: Yellow or gold.

Associated glands/organs: Stomach, gallbladder, pancreas, spleen, adrenals, liver, diaphragm, kidneys, nervous system, muscles.

Possible imbalance: Diabetes, digestive issues, pancreatic issues, eating issues, overweight, underweight, weight loss, excessive hunger, picky eating, food sensitivities, depression, epilepsy, fading newborn syndrome, fears, lack of confidence, immune system issues, obsessive behaviour, training issues, nervousness, shyness, attention seeking and destructive behaviours, over-vocalization, Cushing's disease, Addison's disease, exocrine pancreatic insufficiency (EPI).

🐾 A balanced solar plexus chakra can result in a dog who is confidant, comfortable, personable and cheerful, connected and engaged with others, experiences a well-functioning digestive system from start to finish, is calm and laid-back.

🐾 An imbalanced solar plexus chakra can result in a dog who is a picky eater; experiences vomiting, diarrhoea or constipation; lacks confidence and (sometimes) even the strength or will to live; a dog with a weak immune system; diabetes or other metabolic issues.

Spirit animal: The spirit or totem animal associated with the solar plexus chakra is the lion. The lion relates to strength, patience, cooperation and gentleness. Call in or ask lion energy to come forth to your canine companion to be with her for the purpose of healing her solar plexus chakra.

Ways to stimulate the solar plexus chakra: Spend time with your dog in the sun, encourage them to run while playing or for treats, communicate with them, teach them new things.

Archangel: Jophiel is the archangel associated with the solar plexus chakra. You can call upon Archangel Jophiel to balance your dog's energy related to the solar plexus chakra, and at the same time to release any and all non-beneficial energies to be transmuted by the spiritual realm. Feel free to list any specifics you are aware of as you ask for assistance from the archangels.

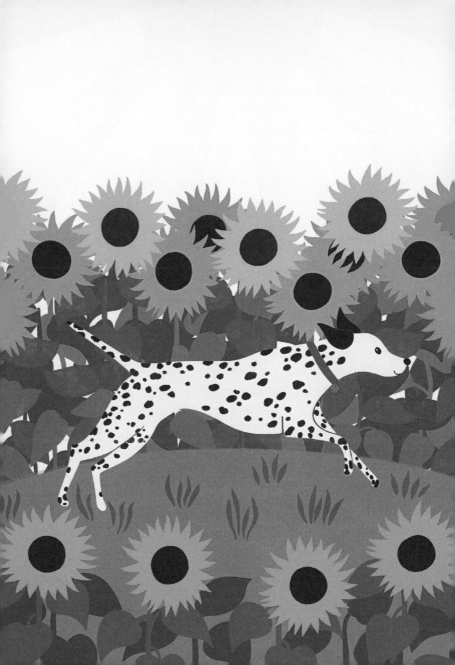

Affirmations: You can create your own affirmation to suit your dog's particular situation or use one of the following:

"[Dog's name] is confident in all situations."

"[Dog's name]'s digestive system functions perfectly."

"[Dog's name] is emotionally engaged with her human and animal friends."

Visualization: If you've determined that the solar plexus chakra is imbalanced, first visualize it as it currently is, and then, on the count of three, visualize it coming into perfect balance. Then visualize "locking it in" to this balanced fashion so that it will stay balanced.

For crystal healing, pendulum dowsing and brain integration: Refer to these sections under the root chakra section (see pages 54–5).

CRYSTALS THAT AID IN HEALING THE SOLAR PLEXUS CHAKRA

Amber	Tiger eye
Citrine	Topaz
Moldavite	Yellow calcite
Sunstone	Yellow fluorite

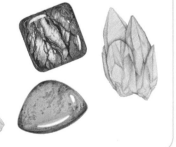

Heart Chakra

Related to both divine and unconditional love, especially the love shared between dogs and their humans, but also the love shared with their animal friends. It is one of the places that connects dogs to their higher power or source energy. A broken heart creates imbalance in this chakra, so it is a chakra that almost always needs balancing in abandoned, abused and rescue dogs. It is the key area for interspecies telepathic communication (also known as animal communication) with humans, as well as communication with others – of their species and others in their household or pack. This chakra energizes the blood and physical body with life force energy.

Location: Centre of the chest, at the heart.

Associated colours: Green or pink.

Associated glands/organs: Heart, thymus, lungs, respiratory system, circulatory system, chest, immune system, front legs and paws.

Possible imbalance: Anger, aggression, broken-hearted, arthritis, anxiety, loneliness for humans or other animals, heart disease, heart murmurs, lung disease, blood disorders, emotional issues, inability to bond, respiratory infection, coughing, stress-related asthma; absorbing energies, emotions, illnesses and non-beneficial energies from humans (or other animals).

🐾 A balanced heart chakra can result in a dog who has a good life, feels loved and offers love freely to both humans and other animal friends, feels energized, enjoys interspecies telepathic communication (animal communication) with her humans.

🐾 An imbalanced heart chakra can result in a dog who has a broken heart from being abandoned, lost or a part of the rescue system; has heart, respiratory or circulatory issues; is anxious, unwilling, displays anger and aggression; failure to thrive.

Spirit animal: The spirit or totem animal associated with the heart chakra is the dolphin. The dolphin relates to love, joy, passion and fertility. Call in or ask dolphin energy to come forth to your canine companion to be with her for the purpose of healing her heart chakra.

Ways to stimulate the heart chakra: Spend time with your dog in nature and with loved ones – human and animal – pet them, communicate with them.

Archangel: Raphael is the archangel associated with the heart chakra. You can call upon Archangel Raphael to balance your dog's energy related to the heart chakra, and at the same time to release any and all non-beneficial energies to be transmuted by the spiritual realm. Feel free to list any specifics you are aware of as you ask for assistance from the archangels.

Affirmations: You can create your own affirmation to suit your dog's particular situation or use one of the following:
"[Dog's name] feels all of the love sent her way."
"[Dog's name]'s negative past is released with grace and replaced with joy."
"[Dog's name]'s life force and vitality are increasing daily."

Visualization: If you've determined that the heart chakra is imbalanced, first visualize it as it currently is, and then, on the count of three, visualize it coming into perfect balance. Then visualize "locking it in" to this balanced fashion so that it will stay balanced.

For crystal healing, pendulum dowsing and brain integration: Refer to these sections under the root chakra section (see pages 54–5).

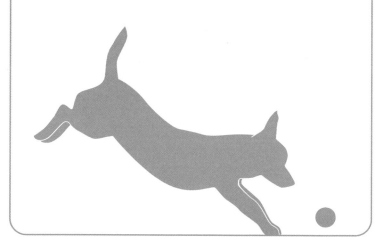

CRYSTALS THAT AID IN HEALING THE HEART CHAKRA

Aventurine

Emerald

Green quartz

Green tourmaline

Kunzite

Pink or green jade

Pink tourmaline

Rose quartz

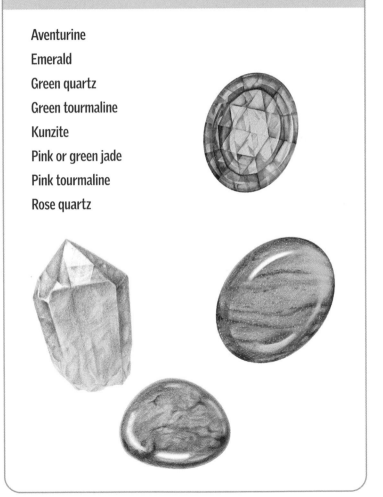

Throat Chakra

Considered to be the communication hub, this chakra is related to all aspects of physical communication and creative expression, especially conscious communication with intent. Self-expression, listening to and interacting with you are also associated with the throat chakra. Truth, clarity, knowledge and wisdom are all traits connected with the throat chakra. Dogs most frequently use their voice to communicate, but any actions used to communicate and express themselves, such as begging, staring or actions based in jealousy or anger are all related to this chakra.

Location: Throat area.

Associated colour: Sky blue.

Associated glands/organs: Throat, thyroid, parathyroid, hypothalamus, mouth, teeth, vocal cords.

Possible imbalance: Depression, excessive or complete lack of vocalization, vocal issues, metabolism, teething, thyroid issues, lack of discernment, knowledge used unwisely, attention-seeking and destructive behaviours, upper respiratory infection, coughing, inappropriate scratching, retaliation, dental issues, stomatitis, inflamed gums, tooth extractions, halitosis.

A balanced throat chakra can result in a dog who is communicative in a balanced and friendly way, interacts with you and others, is happy with her circumstances, is wise, is understanding of attention and devoted to others.

 An imbalanced throat chakra can result in a dog who is depressed, overly demanding or vocal, whiny, urinates or defecates inappropriately, digs holes, has thyroid issues, needs her teeth cleaned.

Spirit animal: The spirit or totem animal associated with the throat chakra is the bear. The bear relates to rhythm, flow, alignment and heeding our inner voice. Call in or ask bear energy to come forth to your canine companion to be with her for the purpose of healing her throat chakra.

Ways to stimulate the throat chakra: Play with your dog, communicate with them, sing to them, play music for them, meditate with them and be creative around or with them.

Archangel: Michael is the archangel associated with the throat chakra. You can call upon Archangel Michael to balance your dog's energy related to the throat chakra, and at the same time to release any and all non-beneficial energies to be transmuted by the spiritual realm. Feel free to list any specifics you are aware of as you ask for assistance from the archangels.

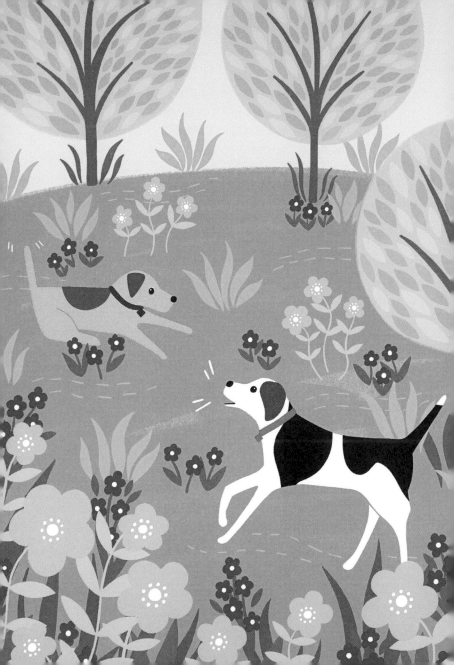

Affirmations: You can create your own affirmation to suit your dog's particular situation or use one of the following:
"[Dog's name] communicates her wishes to me in acceptable ways."
"[Dog's name]'s vocalization habits are perfectly balanced."
"[Dog's name] has a cheerful demeanour."

Visualization: If you've determined that the throat chakra is imbalanced, first visualize it as it currently is, and then, on the count of three, visualize it coming into perfect balance. Then visualize "locking it in" to this balanced fashion so that it will stay balanced.

For crystal healing, pendulum dowsing and brain integration: Refer to these sections under the root chakra section (see pages 54–5).

CRYSTALS THAT AID IN HEALING THE THROAT CHAKRA

Amazonite
Angelite
Aquamarine
Blue lace agate
Celestite
Lapis lazuli
Sodalite
Turquoise

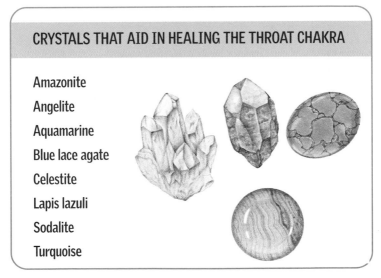

Sensing Chakra

Related to the sensory intake and transmission of sensory information to the brain. In other words, how our canine companions filter and assimilate all experiences that occur, and how they deal with any and all sensory stimuli (seeing, hearing, smelling, touching, feeling and even knowing). But when this chakra is out of balance, even normally occurring circumstances can range from triggering to terrifying. Make sure you check and balance this chakra in any abandoned, lost or rescue dog. The sensing chakra is the reason dogs have heightened sensing ability compared to humans.

Location: Bridge of the nose between the tip of the nose and the eyes.

Associated colour: Silver blue.

Associated glands/organs: Face, nose, eyes, ears, paw pads, whiskers, tail tip.

Possible imbalance: Over- or under-reacting to events, noises, circumstances or training cues; any imbalance of the eyes, ears, nose, tail, etc.; docked tails, clipped whiskers, blindness, deafness, inappropriate elimination, aggression, intolerance, timidity, excessive licking, dislikes nail trimming, excessive foraging – eating plants, flowers or other non-edibles.

🐾 A balanced sensing chakra can result in a dog who is comfortable, confident, calm and trusting, and has a good awareness and perception of her senses, including seeing, hearing, smelling, touching and feeling.

🐾 An imbalanced sensing chakra can result in a dog who is skittish, excitable, fearful, timid; dislikes having her nails trimmed; is lacking in natural sensing and assimilation abilities; forages for non-edibles; or results from being an abandoned, stray or rescue dog.

Spirit animal: The spirit or totem animal associated with the sensing chakra is the turtle. The turtle relates to new opportunities, manifesting, awakening to and connecting with our primal senses. Call in or ask turtle energy to come forth to your canine companion to be with her for the purpose of healing her sensing chakra.

Ways to stimulate the sensing chakra: Meditate, stargaze or watch clouds with your dog; learn about subtle energies from her and work with subtle energies with her; communicate with her.

Archangel: Metatron is the archangel associated with the sensing chakra. You can call upon Archangel Metatron to balance your dog's energy related to the sensing chakra, and at the same time to release any and all non-beneficial energies to be transmuted by the spiritual realm. Feel free to list any specifics you are aware of as you ask for assistance from the archangels.

Affirmations: You can create your own affirmation to suit your dog's particular situation or use one of the following:

"[Dog's name] reacts calmly to normal day-to-day occurrences."

"[Dog's name] releases any and all tendencies to overreact."

"[Dog's name] is becoming more and more tolerant of other dogs and household companions."

Visualization: If you've determined that the sensing chakra is imbalanced, first visualize it as it currently is, and then, on the count of three, visualize it coming into perfect balance. Then visualize "locking it in" to this balanced fashion so that it will stay balanced.

For crystal healing, pendulum dowsing and brain integration: Refer to these sections under the root chakra section (see pages 54–5).

CRYSTALS THAT AID IN HEALING THE SENSING CHAKRA

Angelite

Aquamarine

Blue lace agate

Celestite

Chalcedony

Lapis lazuli

Phantom quartz

Sapphire

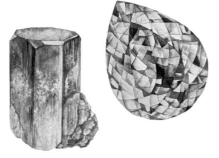

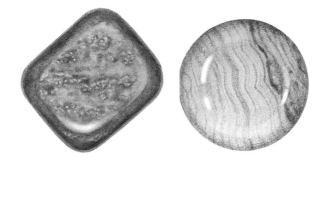

Third Eye Chakra
(Brow Chakra)

Related to psychic insight and universal connection. Self-acceptance, levelheadedness, calmness, ability to focus, soul realization, concentration and devotion are important aspects of this chakra. It is another of the key areas for interspecies telepathic communication (also known as animal communication) with humans, as well as communication with others of their species and others in their household or pack. This chakra is very well developed in most animals, as they are easily in tune, aware and connected unlike many humans. Related to survival instinct, offering dogs the focus and ability required to hunt for their food if required.

Location: Centre of the forehead above the eyes.

Associated colour: Indigo.

Associated glands/organs: Pituitary gland, pineal, ears, left eye, nose, fur, hair, skin.

Possible imbalance: Headaches, depression, boredom, concentration issues, hair loss, hot spots, itching, hearing loss, hyperactivity, post-traumatic pain or stress, allergies, canine acne, dandruff, hormone issues, nervous system, neurological issues, congestion, runny nose, allergies, ear issues including ear mites, eye issues including irritable eyes, conjunctivitis, cataracts.

🐾 A balanced third eye chakra can result in a dog who is accepting, calm, focused, aware, in tune, connected to her surroundings and others, connected psychically, a willing participant in interspecies telepathic communication.

🐾 An imbalanced third eye chakra can result in a dog who is stressed, hyperactive, excitable, disconnected from her surroundings and others, uninterested in interspecies telepathic communication, experiences skin disorders or hair loss.

Spirit animal: The spirit or totem animal associated with the third eye chakra is the eagle. The eagle relates to vision, mysticism, power and healing. Call in or ask eagle energy to come forth to your canine companion to be with her for the purpose of healing her third eye chakra.

Ways to stimulate the third eye chakra: Meditate, stargaze or watch clouds with your dog; communicate with her, focus on bridging the gap between physical knowing and universal truth – conduct esoteric studies in the presence of your dog.

Archangel: Zadkiel is the archangel associated with the third eye chakra. You can call upon Archangel Zadkiel to balance your dog's energy related to the third eye chakra, and at the same time to release any and all non-beneficial energies to be transmuted by the spiritual realm. Feel free to list any specifics you are aware of as you ask for assistance from the archangels.

Affirmations: You can create your own affirmation to suit your dog's particular situation or use one of the following:

"[Dog's name] is calm and accepting."

"[Dog's name] enjoys communication with myself and others."

"[Dog's name] is at one with the Universe and her psychic connection."

Visualization: If you've determined that the third eye chakra is imbalanced, first visualize it as it currently is, and then, on the count of three, visualize it coming into perfect balance. Then visualize "locking it in" in this balanced fashion so that it will stay balanced.

For crystal healing, pendulum dowsing and brain integration: Refer to these sections under the root chakra section (see pages 54–5).

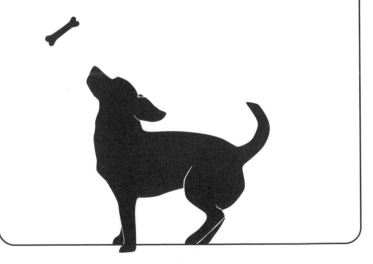

CRYSTALS THAT AID IN HEALING THE THIRD EYE CHAKRA

Azurite
Chalcedony
Iolite
Lapis lazuli
Moonstone
Opal

Pearl
Selenite
Sodalite
Star sapphire
Suglite

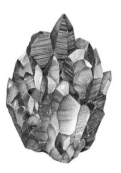

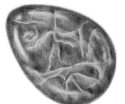

Crown Chakra

Related to the life force connection with the infinite (with God/Goddess, the Universe, spirit). Think of this as the centre responsible for the soul (or essence) of your dog, inhabiting her body. It governs a dog's connection with the world around her and provides access to the vast collective consciousness and universal wisdom, enabling the ability to communicate naturally on subjects far greater than might be expected. This is the chakra of divine wisdom, deep understanding, connection with world around her, selfless service and perception beyond space and time; exactly what you'd hope for from your dog.

Location: Top of the head.

Associated colours: Violet or white.

Associated glands/organs: Cerebral cortex, skull, brain, central nervous system, right eye, pineal gland.

Possible imbalance: Neurological issues, epilepsy, grief, depression, disorientation, fear, headaches, hyperactive, panic attacks, boredom, pining, senility, separation anxiety, stress, tension, sleep issues, training issues, perception of reality, eye issues including irritable eyes, conjunctivitis, cataracts.

🐾 A balanced crown chakra can result in a dog who is relaxed and well-integrated in her body on this earth plane, well-connected to source energy, the spiritual realm and the world around her and able to tap into universal wisdom, aware of and connected to her mission, strong self-healing ability and ability to heal in general.

🐾 An imbalanced crown chakra can result in a dog who suffers the injustices done to her species as a whole, individually as well as through world events and natural disasters; experiences headaches, anxiety, pain or neurological issues.

Spirit animal: The spirit or totem animal associated with the crown chakra is the bee. The bee relates to new choices, fertility, fulfilment and spiritual guidance. Call in or ask bee energy to come forth to your canine companion to be with her for the purpose of healing her crown chakra.

Ways to stimulate the crown chakra: Focus on mutual dreams and intentions; connect to spirit and practise metaphysical studies in the presence of your dog; connect to your mission in the presence of your dog; focus on bridging the gap between physical knowing and universal truth.

Archangel: Gabriel is the archangel associated with the crown chakra. You can call upon Archangel Gabriel to balance your dog's energy related to the crown chakra, and at the same time to release any and all non-beneficial energies to be transmuted by the spiritual realm. Feel free to list any specifics you are aware of as you ask for assistance from the archangels.

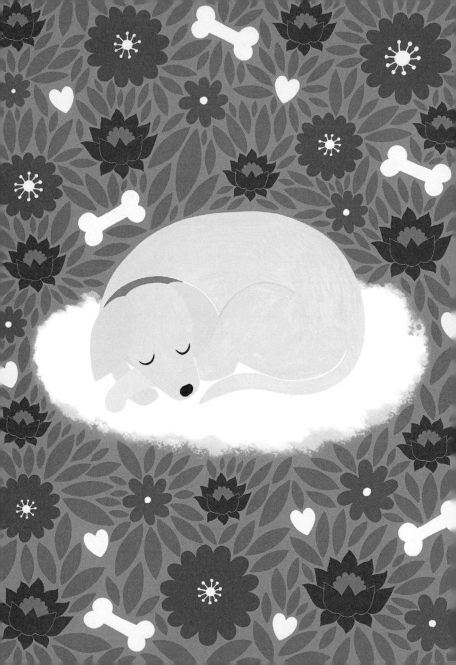

Affirmations: You can create your own affirmation to suit your dog's particular situation or use one of the following:

"[Dog's name] is comfortable in her skin."

"[Dog's name]'s brain and neurological system are fully balanced."

"[Dog's name] has complete access to the collective consciousness and universal wisdom."

Visualization: If you've determined that the crown chakra is imbalanced, first visualize it as it currently is, and then, on the count of three, visualize it coming into perfect balance. Then visualize "locking it in" to this balanced fashion so that it will stay balanced.

For crystal healing, pendulum dowsing and brain integration: Refer to these sections under the root chakra section (see pages 54–5).

CRYSTALS THAT AID IN HEALING THE CROWN CHAKRA

Amethyst	Lepidolite
Diamond	Purple fluorite
Herkimer diamond	Quartz
Lemurian diamond	Violet tourmaline

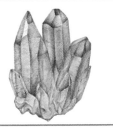

Brachial Chakra

This is a very powerful major energy centre in dogs, relating to connection, transformation and energy flow. This chakra is a central hub from where you can access all of the other chakras, both major and minor, as well as gleaning an entire picture of what is going on in the energy field of your dog. It is another key chakra where dogs and their humans can connect, bond and communicate, and a great chakra to work with to re-establish a weak or lost connection with one another. It is a place from where you can treat the whole body and entire chakra system, and it is recommended as the starting point for any hands-on healing work.

Location: Either side of the lower neck, just in front of the shoulder blade, accessing the brachial plexus nerves.

Associated colour: Black.

Associated glands/organs: Heart, thymus, lungs, respiratory system, circulatory system, chest, front legs and paws.

Possible imbalance: A dog with a brachial chakra that needs balancing can experience almost any imbalance conceivable, especially those related to the head, neck and front portion of the body; a dog suffering from cancer; a dog who dislikes human touch or being picked up, or who mirrors the illnesses of humans. Balance this chakra for any dog being introduced to a new home as well as abandoned, rescue or stray dogs.

🐾 A balanced brachial chakra can result in a dog who is balanced, calm, snuggly; enjoys connection to and the touch of humans; open to transformation; open to new family members, visitors and house sitters; well connected with all of the universal elements: fire, earth, metal, water and wood; all-knowing.

🐾 An imbalanced brachial chakra can result in a dog with imbalanced energy in any area but especially the head, neck and front legs; disconnected emotionally; nervous; dislikes human touch and any kind of deeper connection.

Spirit animal: The spirit or totem animal associated with the brachial chakra is the raven. The raven relates to the circle of life, illumination, magic and mysticism. Ask raven energy to come forth to your canine companion to be with her for the purpose of healing her brachial chakra.

Ways to stimulate the brachial chakra: Any and all of the ways mentioned for all of the other major chakras, depending on the issue; especially focusing on deepening your connection with and interspecies telepathic communication with your dog.

Archangel: All of the archangels (Uriel, Chamuel, Jophiel, Raphael, Michael, Metatron, Zadkiel and Gabriel) are associated with the brachial chakra. Call upon any of them to balance your dog's brachial chakra, and at the same time to release any and all non-beneficial energies. Feel free to list any specifics you are aware of as you ask for assistance from the archangels.

Affirmations: You can create your own affirmation to suit your dog's particular situation or use one of the following:
"[Dog's name]'s energy flows perfectly and harmoniously."
"[Dog's name] easily bonds with myself and other family members."
"[Dog's name] enjoys physical touch."

Visualization: If you've determined that the brachial chakra is imbalanced, first visualize it as it currently is, and then, on the count of three, visualize it coming into perfect balance. Then visualize "locking it in" to this balanced fashion so that it will stay balanced.

For crystal healing, pendulum dowsing and brain integration: Refer to these sections under the root chakra section (see pages 54–5).

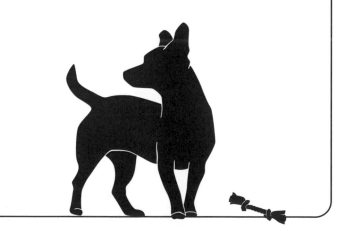

CRYSTALS THAT AID IN HEALING THE BRACHIAL CHAKRA

Black onyx

Black pearl

Black tourmaline

Boji stone

Jet

Shungite

Snowflake obsidian

Tiger eye

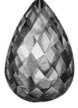

As well as any of the crystals listed to aid in the healing of any of the other major chakras.

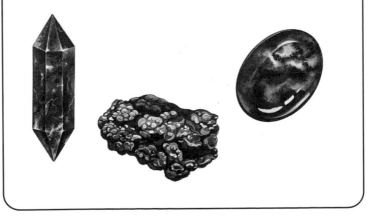

THE MINOR CHAKRAS

Your dog's minor chakras govern and relate to very specific aspects of one or more of her major chakras. It can be advantageous to work with the minor chakras when working on a very specific or specialized sub-issue of a major chakra, as the minor chakras allow us to direct and clear energies specifically related to that issue. For example, the body language chakra is just one aspect of the throat chakra, and when working on the body language chakra, you are directing energy in a more specialized fashion (or direction). In many cases, working on the associated major chakra will handle all your dog's needs, but I wanted to provide options as well as leaving it up to the higher self of your dog to determine which is in her highest and best interest.

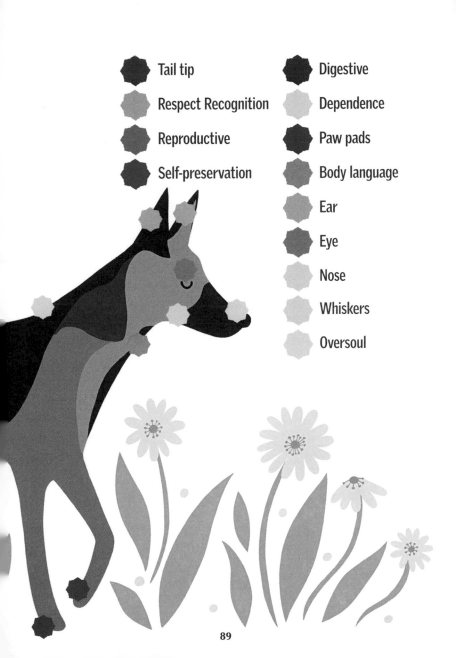

Tail tip

Respect Recognition

Reproductive

Self-preservation

Digestive

Dependence

Paw pads

Body language

Ear

Eye

Nose

Whiskers

Oversoul

Although we haven't provided as many details for each of the minor chakras as we did for the major chakras, please don't presume that they are less important aspects of your dog's energy field. Each of the minor chakras pertains to a vitally important facet of your dog's health and wellbeing, and she will benefit greatly from your attention and healing work related to each of them.

Since the minor chakras are generally lesser-known chakras to most, once you have read the descriptions for each of them, I encourage you to locate them, one by one, on your dog's body – or in her energy field, depending on her sensitivity level. I then recommend that you employ one of the balancing methods listed on pages 42–4 of this book. My suggestion is that you try each of the methods at least once or twice as you work through the balancing process so that you become familiar with, and then embody the feeling of, balancing the chakras energetically. This will aid you in locking in your knowledge of the minor chakras and their locations, as well as the techniques, therefore making it easier for you to remember them in the future.

Self-preservation Chakra

Sub-chakra of the root chakra; see the root chakra for further details (see pages 52–5).

The self-preservation chakra governs the energy that runs down the hind legs of the dog. It is known as the fight-or-flight, adrenal or red-alert state chakra. Its state is representative of the stress or energy drain in dogs living in unharmonious or less than ideal circumstances. This chakra is frequently out of balance in rescue, stray and abused dogs. It is also an issue for dogs living in situations with others (dogs, cats or humans) that they don't get along with.

Location: Hip joint.

Associated colour: Red.

Possible imbalance: Aggression, dominance, bullying, territoriality, resource guarding, intolerance, submissiveness, inappropriate urination or defecation, hip dysplasia, arthritis; fear, anxiety or having suffered from abuse.

Reproductive Chakra

Sub-chakra of the root and sexual progression chakras; see the root chakra (pages 52–5) and sexual progression chakra (pages 56–9) for further details.

The reproductive chakra governs all aspects of reproduction, including heat cycles, natural mating instinct, drive to propagate the species, hormone imbalances, false pregnancies and mammary gland issues.

Location: Reproductive organs.

Associated colour: Red-orange.

Possible imbalance: False pregnancy, breeding issues of all sorts, irregular heat cycles, ovarian cysts, spay/neuter issues, maternal instinct.

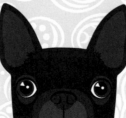

Digestive Chakra

Sub-chakra of the solar plexus chakra; see the solar plexus chakra for further details (see pages 60–3).

Governs all aspects of digestion, including eating issues, weight issues, hunting abilities, excessive foraging and the natural instinct to avoid poisons and other inedible items.

Location: Tip of the liver.

Associated colour: Rust red.

Possible imbalance: Vomiting, diarrhoea, stomach upset, colitis, acid reflux, scavenging, anorexia, ravenous appetite, or a foreign object in the digestive system.

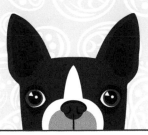

Respect Recognition Chakra

Sub-chakra of the sexual progression chakra; see the sexual progression chakra for further details (see pages 56–9).

Governs territory and social customs beyond the dog's household and family members. Also known as the friend or foe centre.

Location: Spine above internal reproductive organs.

Associated colour: Gold.

Possible imbalance: Over-protective, over-concerned or over-responsible dogs, territorial issues, fear or aggression towards unknown dogs or humans, poor breeding issues (in nature the best genes are deferred to in order to propagate a species) and any other issues related to procreation.

Dependence Chakra

Sub-chakra of the solar plexus chakra; see the solar plexus chakra for further details (see pages 60–3).

The place of independence, trust and obedience with people, and of dominance or submission with other animals.

Location: Underbelly below gallbladder.

Associated colour: Citron yellow.

Possible imbalance: Insecurity, trust issues, training issues, dominance, submissiveness, nervousness and fear.

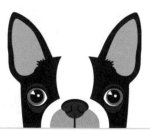

Body Language Chakra

Sub-chakra of the throat chakra; see the throat chakra for further details (see pages 68–71).

Governs behaviour in intentional communication (tail wagging, barking, whining, pawing, smiling, imitating humans). Controls the energy that runs along the spine, down the legs and into the paws.

Location: Behind the throat chakra.

Associated colour: Blue.

Possible imbalance: Excessive vocalization or communication, lack of vocalization or communication, any kind of intentional physical communication such as pawing, staring and other behaviours.

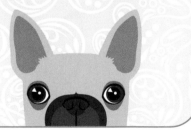

Eye Chakra

Sub-chakra of the sensing chakra; see the sensing chakra for further details (see pages 72–5).

Associated with the sensing chakra and related to any issues pertaining to the eyes and vision.

Location: Eyes.

Associated colours: Violet or lavender.

Possible imbalance: Cataracts, glaucoma, blindness, fading vision, runny eyes, eyelash issues, eye infections and allergies.

Ear Chakra

Sub-chakra of the sensing chakra; see the sensing chakra for further details (see pages 72–5).

Associated with the sensing chakra and related to any issues pertaining to the ears and hearing.

Location: Base of the ears.

Associated colours: Aqua or blue.

Possible imbalance: Ear infections, hearing issues, deafness, ear mites, rhinitis and allergies.

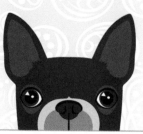

Nose Chakra

Sub-chakra of the sensing chakra; see the sensing chakra for further details (see pages 72–5).

Associated with the sensing chakra and related to any issues pertaining to the nose and sense of smell (a dog's sense of smell is greater than a cat's and is said to be 40 times greater than a human's).

Location: Tip of the nose.

Associated colour: Silver blue.

Possible imbalance: Allergies, sinus infections, sensitivity, lack of smell, picky eater, respiratory issues.

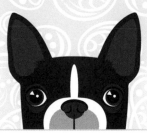

Whiskers Chakra

Sub-chakra of the sensing chakra; see the sensing chakra for further details (see pages 72–5).

Associated with the sensing chakra and related to any issues pertaining to the whiskers.

Location: Face beside the mouth.

Associated colour: Silver blue.

Possible imbalance: Infection, whisker fatigue, clipped or missing whiskers due to injury, issues related to face, mouth, teeth, gums and tongue.

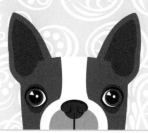

Paw Pads Chakra

Sub-chakra of the sensing chakra; see the sensing chakra for further details (see pages 72–5).

Associated with the sensing chakra and related to any issues pertaining to the paw pads.

Location: Bottom of the feet.

Associated colour: Ruby red.

Possible imbalance: Dogs with amputations, nail clipping concerns or any other issues of the paw pads.

Tail Tip Chakra

Sub-chakra of the sensing and root chakras; see the sensing chakra (pages 72–5) and the root chakra (pages 52–5) for further details.

Associated with the sensing and root chakras and related to any issues pertaining to the tail tip.

Location: Tip of the tail (if the tail has been cropped, it is where the tail would have ended).

Associated colour: Dark red.

Possible imbalance: Dogs with docked tails, amputations, abrasions, infections and any other tail issues.

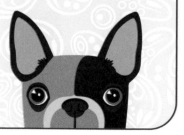

Oversoul Chakra
(Transpersonal Point Chakra)

Sub-chakra of the third eye and crown chakras; see the third eye chakra (pages 76–9) and the crown chakra (pages 80–3) for further details.

The connection of an individual dog to their higher self, spirit and the Universe, as well as their connection to their soul group; also known as an oversoul.

Location: Base of the skull or above the crown chakra.

Associated colours: White or silver.

Possible imbalance: Any imbalance related to the third eye or crown chakra, especially those connected with the unseen realms, telepathy and psychic insight. With this chakra, I usually wait until the chakra comes up to be balanced and just trust that it is in divine order.

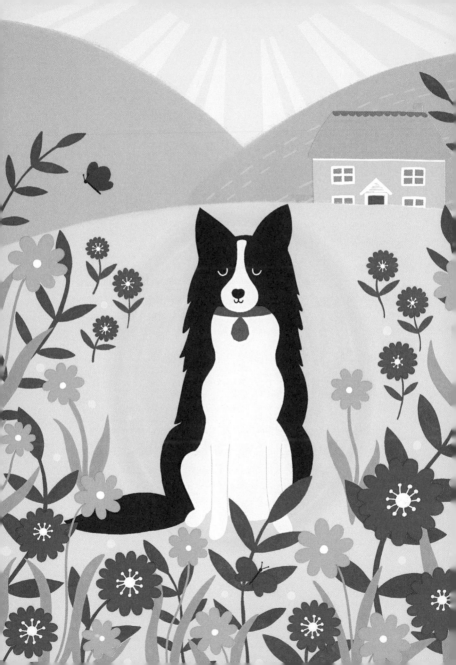

PART THREE
WHOLE-BODY HEALING

The tools and techniques featured in this section work with the body as an integrated whole to facilitate healing in the energy field and therefore the chakras. They include the energy techniques of Reiki, crystal healing, colour therapy and the use of flower essences and gem elixirs.

SIX SIMPLE ENERGY TECHNIQUES

Since dogs are so receptive to energy, sometimes even the seemingly smallest techniques can have a big impact. Whether your canine companion needs balance in a specific area related to one of her chakras or just seems a little "off" and you are having trouble determining the reason, a tiny energy shift can clear an imbalance and promote health and wellbeing.

The grounding exercise mentioned in Part One is always the simplest and best place to start, followed by the brain integration technique also in Part One (see pages 32–3 and 42). From there, you can try one (or more) of these six simple energy exercises. Some are for specific healing purposes and others are intended to be performed daily as maintenance, so use your judgement and remember to attune to your canine companion's wishes and preferences.

Pure Positive Intention

It may sound like a small thing, but as mentioned earlier, positive intention can go a long way towards balancing and healing your canine companion's energy field and chakras. Setting your intention related to the health and wellbeing of your canine friend is an easy technique that can be done daily and can have a tremendous effect.

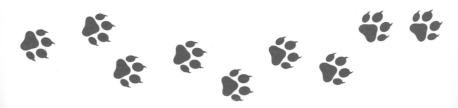

Feng Shui

Feng shui, the Chinese art of placement, helps to harmonize and create balance with the natural world, which is very important for dogs, especially those living indoors. Having a well-organized home clear of clutter – both physically and energetically – can help restore energy flow and keep your dog's energy balanced. Keeping your house tidy and dust-free as well as clearing cobwebs and opening windows will promote a smoother energy flow. Clearing your home and your dog's space energetically, including the corners or rooms where energy can tend to get trapped, can be done by ringing Tibetan tingsha bells, smudging with sage, clapping your hands to break up the energy or using an energy cleansing spray. Any and all of these methods can help prevent energy from collecting there and will also encourage a healthy flow.

Sacred Symbols

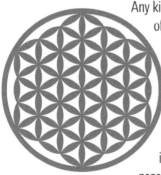

Any kind of sacred geometry, such as the flower of life or a similar sacred symbol, can bring a positive shift to the energy of your canine companion. A good way to utilize the symbol is to print it out, laminate it and place it near your dog's favourite sleeping spot. You can write positive affirmations on it that you want to infuse into your dog's energy field, such as love, peace, harmony, joy, etc.

Connecting All Parts

Helping your dog become more aware of her entire body and energy field can calm and relax her, especially for dogs with abuse or abandonment issues. To do this, simply touch her all over, including her legs, paws and other areas, with the intention of bringing her awareness to all of her body parts. Pay attention to what your dog likes, from light touch to massage, and proceed gently to calm her aura.

Ear Pressure Points

Working on the numerous pressure points on your dog's ears can relieve a wide variety of issues, from aches and pains to digestive disorders and anxiety. This technique can feel comforting to your dog, like a massage. Taking your index finger, curl it sideways inside the base of the ear with your thumb on the outside. From the base of the ear, run your finger and thumb up to the top edge with slight pressure. Repeat, working your way across until you've covered the entire ear, and then do the same on the other ear.

Lifesaving Acupressure Point

If your dog has a negative reaction to an insect bite or sting – or experiences trauma or injury – this acupressure point can potentially save her life by reviving consciousness and re-centring her energy field. This can be done if your dog faints or has a seizure – or on the way to the veterinarian in an emergency. Known as GV-26, the point is located where your dog's nose meets her mouth. Sited on the governing meridian of the energy field, GV-26 is important for any animal lover to know. To stimulate this point, take the pad of your thumb and push hard – in an emergency, you can even use your fingernail.

REIKI

Reiki, based in balance and a profoundly deep connection with another, is a beautiful, peaceful healing space you can share with your dog – one that will forever change you and the bond you share. Often referred to as a healing modality, it is truly so much more than that. Reiki is a system; an energetic essence; a gateway to connection and to who you are at your very essence. Those who practise Reiki are referred to as practitioners, not healers, since they don't manipulate the healing of others but rather invite and allow it.

Created by Mikao Usui, Reiki is an ancient Japanese healing practice or energy system based on compassionate intention, one that works brilliantly to offer the space or opening for healing. The Japanese word "reiki" translates to "spiritual energy" or "universal life-force energy". When you are "attuned" by a Reiki master to the concept and energy of Reiki, you then become a conduit with the ability to channel universal life-force energy effortlessly. An attunement is the ceremonial initiation or passing on of Reiki information from master to student, reminding students of their innate connection to spirit. Being attuned to Reiki by a master is a requirement for those wishing to practise Reiki.

How Reiki Can Help

Reiki can help with any issue you can think of, whether it be physical, emotional, mental or spiritual. Dogs can benefit greatly from a Reiki session even when they seem to be in perfect health. It's even helpful to aid a dog in passing from the physical to the spiritual realm, as any being can use help, compassion and supportive energy for that process. If you are concerned about your dog's health or you're worried and fearful about a diagnosis, use the precepts below and muster up the self-discipline to move into your heart space. Lay any troublesome feelings aside, replacing them with new thoughts of your dog as a divine, healthy and whole being, fully embodying her pure inner light.

The Five Reiki Precepts

Usui established a set of five foundational precepts that all Reiki practitioners and teachers are encouraged to adopt.

The Reiki Precepts

1. Just for today, do not worry.

2. Just for today, do not anger.

3. Just for today, be humble.

4. Just for today, be honest.

5. Just for today, be compassionate towards yourself and others.

Self-healing

Practitioners can use Reiki healing not only to work on others, but also to work on themselves for their own health and wellbeing. In fact, working on self-healing is a prerequisite for anyone offering Reiki to others.

Based on the concept that all living beings possess divine power and wisdom within, a Reiki session works within your dog's energy field to improve her health, creating balance and therefore improving the quality of her life. Reiki has been known to soothe, heal, relax and energize a dog, depending on what they need most in the moment. Reiki is a fabulous method of healing for our canine companions, who – for the most part – love to soak up this healing energy.

Reiki, in its beginning, involved the "laying on of hands" as well as distance work, which is of great benefit for dogs who may be timid, fearful, confined to a veterinary hospital or in too much pain to tolerate hands-on work. Distance Reiki for animals is an option that has gained popularity in recent years and has evolved into a highly respectful modality that deeply honours the canine recipient, resulting in a prayerful, meditative union for the highest and best good of all. It is now widely considered the preferred way to offer healing to animals.

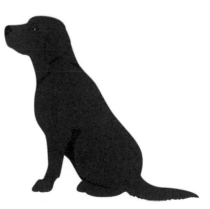

A Reiki Session

Many but not all dogs enjoy hands-on Reiki, so always let the dog decide. If you are doing hands-on Reiki, always aim to be as unobtrusive and non-invasive as possible. Use a soft, relaxed approach. There is no need to move your hands to various positions as you may have been taught unless your dog signifies that she wants you to do so. There is also no need to focus on energy flowing from your hands to your dog; in fact, it's best if you don't.

1 Before you begin a Reiki treatment, close your eyes and take a couple of deep, cleansing breaths. Enter a form of prayerful meditation, centring yourself, bringing the palms of your hands together in front of your upper chest, and spend a few moments connecting to the Reiki energy while clearing your mind of everything else.

Place yourself approximately 5–10 ft (1.5–3 m) away from your dog, and then greet and ask for permission to do a Reiki treatment. At the same time, set your intention for the session. Release any attachments or expectations you have related to whether the dog will want to engage physically with you, how the dog will receive the energy or whether she will walk away, as none of this matters. Only offer hands-on treatment if the dog comes towards you or leans into your hands.

 Once you begin the Reiki treatment, simply let the flow guide you. Offer the treatment for approximately 30–60 minutes whether the dog stays with you or not, and at the conclusion, thank the dog for her connection and conclude the session.

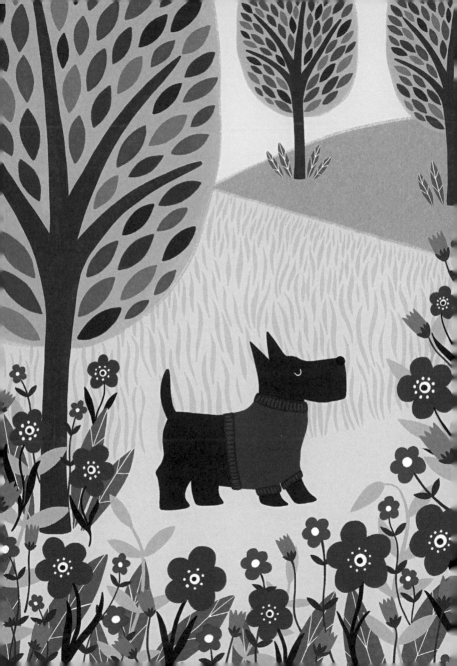

COLOUR THERAPY

Colour therapy, also known as chromotherapy, is a form of healing that uses a combination of colour and light to treat certain physical, emotional and mental health conditions. In the past, this was done by shining a light bulb through a theatrical colour gel (of the desired colour for the particular issue requiring healing) to create coloured light to treat your dog's ailments. In more recent years, coloured light wands, specialized torches and home-healing kits have emerged, making the application of colour therapy easier. Our dogs' cells generate vital energy from light; in healing work, light and colour combined can balance and replenish vibrant energy in our dogs in a non-invasive way.

Working with Colour

One of the ways to work with colour is to determine the priority chakra requiring balancing and then apply the colour of that chakra (see Part Two) to the chakra and/or the entire body. For example: for a digestive ailment, the associated major chakra is the solar plexus chakra and the colour is yellow, so you could bathe your dog or your dog's solar plexus chakra in yellow light.

Another example is if you notice your dog seems very ungrounded, which can be common after any traumatic event. Since the chakra associated with groundedness is the root chakra, you could bathe your dog or your dog's root chakra in red-coloured light. This can be done for any traits related to one of your dog's chakras – or just to balance the chakra alone if you feel or have determined that it needs balancing, but you don't currently recognize any outward signs of imbalance. The chart of colours and their properties on the following page provides some of the numerous mental and psychological traits associated with each colour.

Important Notes

🐾 As with most healing modalities, it's important that your colour therapy work be set up in such a way that your dog is allowed to come and go at will and not have it forced upon them constantly.

🐾 I also caution you not to shine coloured light directly in your dog's eyes, as some sensitive beings may have issues with this that would counteract the healing process.

Colours and Their Properties

Red:	Courage, stimulation, strength, groundedness
Orange:	Self-confidence, resilience, upliftment
Yellow:	Mental alertness, optimism, playfulness
Green:	Peace, balance, emotional calm
Turquoise:	Tranquillity, restoration, refreshment
Blue:	Calming, contentment, confidence
Violet:	Change, transformation, accelerated vibrations
Purple:	Soothing, calms emotions, creativity
Indigo:	Purpose, inspiration, protection
Magenta:	Mental and emotional balance, acceptance, confidence
Pink:	Happiness, joy, sensitivity

How to Use Colour

To perform colour therapy properly, resulting in ideal outcomes, you need the right equipment that combines colour and light, which can come at a considerable cost. Many still wishing to work with colour but not willing or able to invest in this type of equipment take a more casual approach and simply introduce more of the relevant colour into their dog's environment. This can be done in the following ways.

- Physically apply coloured fabric to the particular chakra you want to balance, as well as the rest of the body, perhaps in the form of a T-shirt or coat.

- Lay a piece of coloured fabric – of the colour of the chakra you want to balance, or the trait you want to expand – over your dog's bed or sleeping areas.

- Use coloured leads and collars.

- Provide toys in the colour of the chakra you want to balance.

- Provide food and water bowls of the colour of the chakra you want to balance.

- If appropriate, provide food (for example, blueberries) of the colour of the chakra you want to balance.

- Paint the room the colour of the chakra you want to balance.

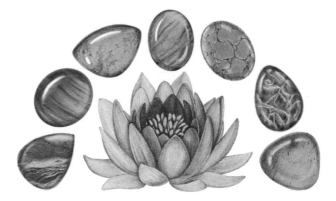

CRYSTAL HEALING

This technique uses crystals and other stones to heal, balance and protect. Crystals encourage positive, healing energy to flow into the body and displace negative, harmful energy.

What Are Crystals?

Crystals and gemstones are enchanted gifts from the Earth that can promote extraordinary healing in the energy field as well as in the chakras – in both humans and animals. Since canines possess a natural receptivity, crystals work well to draw to themselves the precise energies they require to heal. Crystals are formed naturally in the Earth, and the term "crystal" refers to any precious gem, mineral, stone, fossil or resin that has a measurable charge and produces an electrical pulse.

Important Notes

🐾 It is my preference (and your dog's), especially when working with sensitive animals, that your crystal healing work be set up in such a way that they be allowed to come and go from the crystal energy and not have it forced upon them at all times.

🐾 Certain crystals, including malachite, cinnabar and peacock ore, are toxic. Prevent your dog from licking or mouthing these stones, and even better, *avoid using these stones with dogs*.

🐾 Always make sure the crystals you use are large enough not to be ingested by any animal or small child in the household.

🐾 Crystal healing is not meant to replace veterinary care.

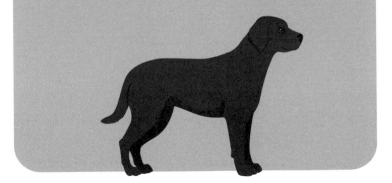

How Crystal Healing Works

Each crystal has a specific vibrational frequency and amplitude, which reverberates or resonates with and attracts the energies of certain qualities or traits in your dog. Crystal healing is a non-invasive healing technique that works on all levels of consciousness: physical, emotional, mental and spiritual.

Clearing crystals

Before you begin using crystals with your dog, it's important to clear the energy of the crystal. This can be done by leaving the crystal out in the sunlight or moonlight, by using smoke from a smudge stick or with your intention.

Programming crystals

A crystal can be programmed for a specific use simply by placing it in your hand. Then, while you are in a healing state, assign it a particular job or task; ask it to help a particular animal with a particular situation or issue. This can be done by saying the words either out loud, or silently, inside your head.

For example, hold a piece of blue lace agate (a cooling stone) in your hand and ask it to help calm your dog's excessive vocalization and demanding nature. Then place it in your dog's environment and watch it work.

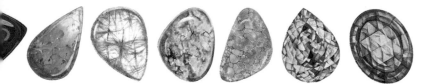

Ways to Work with Crystals and Your Dog

Place some crystals in her space. Affix a crystal pendant onto your dog's collar, zip a crystal into her bedding or place one under her favourite chair.

❧

Give your dog a crystal massage. Massage her with a crystal wand or other smooth, tumbled stone. This can be done on the body or in the aura.

❧

Place a crystal in her water bowl (make sure it is large enough not to be ingested by any animal in the household). This will infuse her water (and thus her) with the properties of the crystal.

❧

Create a crystal layout, spread around a stationary animal or at a favourite sunning spot where your dog loves to nap.

❧

Send the frequency of a particular healing crystal to your dog (similar to the technique you learned in Part Two when sending colour to the chakra).

Use this statement: "[Dog's name], receive [name of crystal] perfectly now, on all levels, all dimensions, all aspects known and unknown, now and for all time."

🐾

Wear crystals yourself as jewellery when you are around your canine friend.

🐾

Protect her space. This can be done by placing four crystal points in the corner of a crate, kennel, dog bed or your canine companion's favourite part of the house, with the intention that they are for protection. Clear quartz is most commonly used for this purpose.

🐾

Crystals can be used intentionally to add or remove energy from your dog or puppy. It's beneficial to add energy to a weak dog or puppy who is not thriving, but in the case of an animal with a lot of heat and inflammation present, such as in the case of an elderly dog with arthritis, removing energy will serve her better.

Increasing and Decreasing Energy

To send energy into an area:

🐾 Hold a clear quartz crystal with a point on one end, 6–12 in (15–30 cm) away from your dog, with the point towards the problem area.

🐾 Then circle clockwise as you move the crystal closer and closer to the area you are treating while setting the intention to add energy and vitality.

To remove energy from an area, do the exact opposite:

🐾 Hold a clear quartz crystal with a point on one end, 1 in (2.5 cm) or so away from your dog, with the tip pointing away from the problem area (but not directly at you).

🐾 Then circle anti-clockwise as you move the crystal further and further away from the area you are treating while setting the intention to remove energy and inflammation.

🐾 You can place the pointed end of a crystal on each side of a problem area and ask the crystal to increase the energy in that area or to clear an energy blockage. Don't rely on this if your dog has eaten a foreign object; it only works for energy blockages.

The Four Master Healers

There are four master healer crystals that can be used for any and all conditions, at any point on the body: clear quartz, rose quartz, amethyst and smoky quartz. These are great crystals to have in your collection.

Let's look at some of the other crystals that can be used for a variety of canine issues. Once you've familiarized yourself with crystal work, you can find the crystals that resonate specifically with your dog's issues in the box below.

Crystals for Dogs

Amethyst: Soothes fears and stresses, calms an anxious dog, reduces pain and inflammation.

Black tourmaline: Protects against negative energy, helps with stress and imbalanced hormones.

Blue lace agate: Anti-inflammatory and cooling. Good for demanding, vocal or hungry dogs.

Chrysoprase: Aids the digestive system. Deeply calming, this stone can help heal separation anxiety and grief.

Citrine: Good for emotional, sensory overload. Boosts the immune system. Any of the yellow stones can be used for issues of the bladder, urinary tract and kidneys.

Copper: Can be used for purification or arthritic conditions, as for humans.

Covellite: Can be used for any serious illness requiring detoxification.

Emerald: Calms and soothes the nerves, boosts confidence in submissive dogs, purifies the system.

Herkimer diamond: Enhances animal communication, releases stress and cleanses the aura.

Jadeite jade: Calms aggression and helps dogs settle into new environments.

Jet: A resin used as a protective talisman since the Stone Age. Grounding and useful in the breaking of negative patterns.

Lapis lazuli: Can be used for respiratory issues, detoxifying, enhancing the energy flow, and to boost the energy.

Peridot: Enhances energy and vitality, encourages harmony in the pack and cleanses toxins.

Rhodolite garnet: Rebalances chakras after shock, repairs aura damage and facilitates the healing of wounds and injuries.

Rose quartz: The crystal of joy and unconditional love. Good for animals that are abused, abandoned, or neglected. It's also good for dogs that have to tolerate something they'd rather not. This is one of my favourite go-to crystals.

Ruby: Heals loneliness and loss, boosts interest in life and brings forth confidence, light and joy.

Selenite: Clears energy blocks; promotes peace and calming. One of the best crystals for help in the treatment of any type of cancer.

Smoky quartz: Grounds, calms, releases stress and nervousness. One of my favourite go-to crystals.

Turquoise: A great healer stone that can also be used for protection, tissue regeneration or as a systemic tonic.

Chakra Healing Crystal Layouts or Grids

You can create a crystal healing layout (often called a grid) for your dog by positioning crystals around her as follows. If your crystals are terminated (have a point at one end), be sure to place them pointing either towards your dog or away from your dog, as suggested below. I don't recommend using double-terminated crystals with points at each end for these grids, but it is fine to use non-terminated crystals.

The Rose Quartz Crystal Layout

Choose a crystal that aids in healing the chakra you wish to work on (from the lists in Part Two); for example, from the heart chakra list, I chose rose quartz. In the previous section, you can see the properties of some of the crystals (which may help you in choosing). The properties of rose quartz are joy, unconditional love and support for abused, abandoned or neglected dogs – and so much more.

You will need eight pieces of rose quartz to position around your dog. If you wish to add energy to your dog's heart chakra, place the pointed (or terminated) ends of the crystals towards your dog. If you wish to reduce energy to your dog's heart chakra, place the pointed (or terminated) ends of the crystals away from your dog. This decision is up to you, but look to your dog to let you know which she prefers.

You can also use one of the four master healer crystals (see page 124) to work on any chakra.

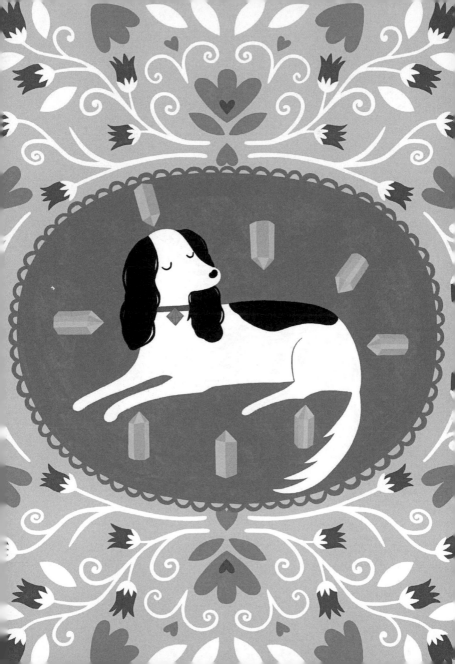

The Clear Quartz Layout

A simple crystal healing layout using clear quartz crystal points can be used to boost your dog's energy or heal a particular injury, illness or wound. You will need three pieces of single terminated clear quartz to position around the area you wish to work on – for example, the face or a paw. This layout can be placed around your dog's bed at night to aid in recovery.

FLOWER ESSENCES AND GEM ELIXIRS

Both flower essences and gem elixirs contain the energy of the plant or stone from which they are derived. These can then be used to bring forth positive effects or treat particular issues.

What Is a Flower Essence?

All living beings have a consciousness, and that also includes flowers. For nearly a century, flower essences have provided powerful, vibrational energy that heals humans and animals alike.

The specific life-force pattern of the flower is contained in its vibrational frequency, and this is the purpose behind creating flower essences. The vibrational and energetic frequencies of the flower are captured in spring water and preserved, often with a type of pure alcohol like vodka. When the essence is applied topically or taken internally, it awakens certain qualities in the human or animal taking it, drawing forth desired traits or positive attributes and encouraging emotional balance.

The history of flower essences

Flower essences were developed in England in the 1930s by Dr Edward Bach, a physician and researcher who set out to harness the power of flowers for healing and wellbeing. Bach Flower Remedies were originally developed for humans, but they have since been found to be incredibly helpful for animals as well – especially since animals' energy systems are less complicated. Dogs are closer to flowers, both physically and energetically, and thus they respond well to flower essences. Through the process of absorbing and embodying the vibrational frequency of the flower, your dog can heal physically, emotionally and mentally, in a number of ways.

Since flower essences are completely fragrance-free and non-toxic, they are perfectly safe and ideal to use with your dog. Unlike essential oils, with which they are often confused and which contain chemical constituents that can be toxic to animals, flower essences are completely safe and have no known side effects. Flower essences won't interfere with medications, so they integrate easily with both holistic and allopathic medicines.

What Is a Gem Elixir?

A gem elixir is made in a very similar way to a flower essence. Instead of a flower, a crystal is chosen and soaked in spring water to capture the vibrational frequency of the crystal in the water. Just as with flowers, different crystals offer different frequencies, energies and benefits through the gem elixir. Also, gem elixirs are equally safe and beneficial to both people and animals.

How to Select Flower Essences and Gem Elixirs

When choosing gem elixirs and flower essences, it's helpful to note that both have no harmful effect on those who do not need them. Indeed, it is recommended that all animals and humans in the household take the same group of essences to integrate and balance all of the energies and produce an environment of harmony. Very often, our animal companions are absorbing energies and emotions from the people in their family, so this can help to clear up any sources of their imbalance.

With this in mind, you can use methods such as dowsing or muscle testing to match the essence to the person and/or dog energetically. I have found these to be the best methods, but there are others that work just as well. You can choose a flower essence for yourself and your dog by determining which flower you are drawn to strongly, or you can also look at your dog's personality and temperament and find an essence that matches based on the essence description (you can look this up online or in books, charts, etc., and also see pages 136–7). Focus on the traits you'd like your dog to release – traits like rigidity or persistence – as well as the positive ones you'd like to restore or strengthen.

When selecting flower essences, you can pick as many as five or six at a time. As mentioned above, it is not harmful to select the wrong remedy; if one is not needed, it cause your dog any ill-effects. However, too many remedies at once will be less effective than fewer well-chosen ones, so try to tune in to your inner self and follow where it leads you for you and your dog. Then, trust your dog to let you know what is and isn't working for her.

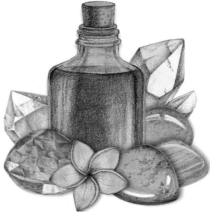

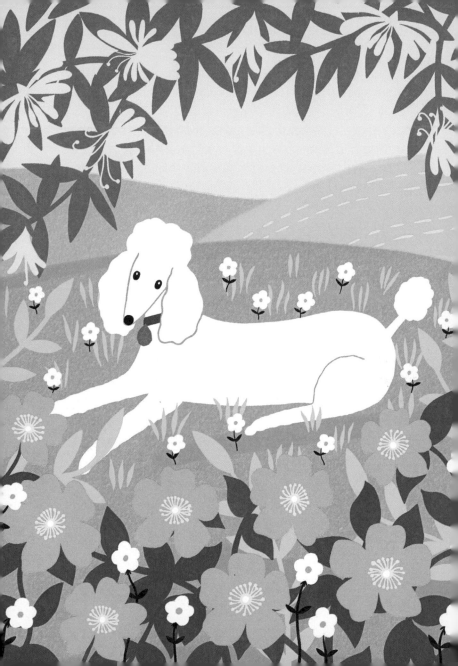

Ways to Administer Flower Essences and Gem Elixirs

The best way to administer flower essences is in your dog's water. Add 2–4 drops of the essence to each bowl of water. Having multiple dogs (and other animal companions) sharing one water bowl is fine. For humans, since it's recommended that we take the same essences as our canine friends, a few drops may be put directly under the tongue or in a glass of water and sipped at least four times a day – more often is even better.

For ease of dispensing a number of flower essences at one time, you can make what's known as a stock bottle, which is a blend of various essences in a clean 1-oz (25-ml) glass bottle with a dropper. You can do this by adding 10–20 drops of each essence and filling it the rest of the way with spring water. Squirt a dropperful into your dog's mouth four times a day (with a plastic dropper for safety), or empty the dropper into her water bowl as described above. Stock bottles must be kept in the refrigerator and will last up to 30 days without contamination. Please note that some dogs prefer not to have the essences squirted into their mouths and it's best to respect their wishes, as adding additional stress will defeat the objective of the healing process (or goal).

Flower essences can also be applied topically to your dog – preferably in a spot where there is no fur, such as on the paw pads, around the muzzle or on the ears. The shoulders or back (part the hair first) are often the easiest. This is particularly recommended for dogs (usually those who get water through a raw food diet) that don't drink frequently enough to ingest the essences four times a day.

As each flower essence or gem elixir has its own unique energy, it is very important to approach giving your dog flower essences or gem elixirs with a positive intention and prayerful ritual when offering them to her. Be decisive and intentional on how you want them to help your animal companion with their healing, respecting the nature spirits involved and the healing power of the essences, and say your prayer or declaration that it will be so.

How to Use Flower Essences and Gem Elixirs in Chakra Healing

When you have a specific trait or behaviour that you're trying to heal in your dog's chakras, it can be useful to own a flower essence guide or pamphlet. For example, if your dog exhibits fear, which is associated with the root chakra, you can look up "fear" in your guide and discover which essence addresses it. If you look up the Bach Flower Remedies, you will see that mimulus, aspen and rock rose are the ideal remedies for fear. You can read about each of the essences and decide whether you feel it's best to give your dog just one or two, or all three together.

If your dog has been rescued, there's a good chance she has several traits that need healing, such as fear (as mentioned above); feeling overwhelmed, discouraged or hopeless; despair, shock or trauma. These traits can have an impact on several of your dog's chakras. If you look up the Bach Flower Remedies for these traits, you will see that their remedies are elm, gentian, gorse, Star of Bethlehem and the fear remedies listed opposite.

You can then give your dog these four essences, plus one or two of the remedies for fear. You can give these to her all together, or another option would be to choose the ones that seem to be needed the most at the time, based on the descriptions in your guide. You can give your dog those for at least four weeks, and then once you've seen some benefit, switch and give her the rest of them.

These are just a few examples of ways you can administer flower essences or gem elixirs – use your intuition and take guidance from your dog, and be ready to listen for clues on how she's responding. Bear in mind that there are many makers of flower essences and gem elixirs with numerous remedies in their catalogues. Therefore, there are far too many to list here; I suggest doing some research and finding one that works for you and your dog on your healing journey together.

TIP: Always store flower essences in a cool, dry place away from sunlight and harmful frequencies like the microwave, as they may have a negative effect on them.

Common Issues in Dogs and Related Flower Essence Recipes

The following remedy suggestions are based on the 38 Bach Flower Remedies.

Accidents: Centaury, Rescue Remedy

Adapting to change: Walnut

Aggression: Beech, holly, vine

Barking (excessive): Chicory, heather

Biting: Chicory, holly

Confusion: Walnut, wild oat

Distress: Agrimony, cherry plum, crab apple, Walnut

Dominance: Beech, rock water, vine

Epilepsy: Cherry plum

Fear: Aspen, mimulus, rock rose

Grief: Star of Bethlehem, Rescue Remedy

Hopelessness: Gentian, gorse

Incontinence: Cherry plum, crab apple

Jealousy: Holly

Licking (constant): Centaury, crab apple, white chestnut

Maliciousness: Holly, willow

Nervousness: Aspen, mimulus, Rescue Remedy

Over-concern: Chicory, red chestnut

Pain (chronic): Agrimony, impatiens

Panic: Aspen, cherry plum, rock rose, Rescue Remedy

Restlessness: Mimulus, white chestnut

Sensitivity: Beech

Shock and trauma: Agrimony, clematis, scleranthus, Star of Bethlehem, Rescue Remedy

Shyness: Aspen, mimulus

Territoriality: Rock water, vine

Whining: Heather

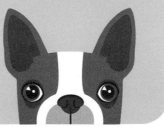

CONCLUSION

It is my hope that the techniques and information within this book will help you when working with your dog for healing and wellbeing. While this book is by no means exhaustive, it should give you and your dog a foundation to work with on your (and her) healing journey. I wish you the best as you proceed, and I always love to hear feedback from my readers and students, so please feel free to share on my website or social media. On the following pages, you will find additional information and resources should you wish to further your study. Enjoy the new and/or deeper connection you have with your canine companion!

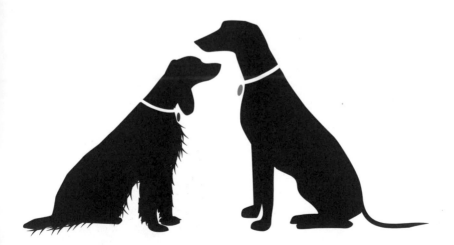

ABOUT THE CONTRIBUTORS

Lynn McKenzie is an expert in the animal intuitive and energy healing fields with over 30 years of experience. Through her signature Animal Energy® Certification Training programme in Sedona, Arizona, Lynn has built a global reputation, helping others identify, foster and embody their inherent gifts. She also offers programmes on spiritual growth, personal transformation, psychic development, clairvoyance mastery and chakra healing (see overleaf). She is the author of *Bark, Neigh, Meow: Awaken to the Transformative Wisdom of Your Companion Animal to Activate Your Soul's Highest Calling.* Visit her at LynnMcKenzie.com.

Painter and maker by trade, **Sian Summerhayes** founded her art business as an extension of her personal practice. With a love for painting original pieces and creating prints, Sian's bright and busy style has naturally evolved to products and decorative homewares. Inspired by the local Cotswold countryside and homely cottage life in rural England, Sian's work brings charm and colour to the home through her trademark depictions of wild flowers, foliage, birds and animals in pretty scenes. Visit her at siansummerhayes.com.

RESOURCES FOR READERS

Now that you are equipped with this information, you may want to go deeper on your healing journey with your dog and expand your knowledge even further.

There are two free resources that will help you open to deeper healing and connection with your canine companions as well as with every aspect of your life.

1. Making the Heart Connection with Your Animal Companions
This training course will help you open even further to deeper connections with your dogs as well as with every aspect of your life. It's a six-part audio series with a workbook and webinar.
https://lynnmckenzie.com/training/

2. How to Master Animal Communication
This is a 90-minute webinar that covers: the three paths to animal communication mastery and how to know which is the best and easiest path for you; the number-one skill you must master to expand your animal communication and feel 100 per cent confident in your abilities; the key ingredient to confidently understanding your animal companions so you always know what they truly want; and the animal communication energy secret that is often missed but instantly makes you feel closer to your animal companions.
www.AnimalEnergyCertification.com

Lynn McKenzie offers in-depth training programmes and home study courses on a variety of topics to help you in the areas of healing, animal communication, psychic development and clairvoyance mastery, which you can learn more about on the website, LynnMcKenzie.com. If you feel called to deepen your connection and explore a new path and calling, take a look here.

BIBLIOGRAPHY

Books

Ted Andrews, *The Animal-wise Tarot*, Dragonhawk Publishing, 1999.

Margrit Coates, *Healing for Horses*, Rider, 2001.

Helen Graham and Gregory Vlamis, *Bach Flower Remedies for Animals*, Findhorn Press, 1999.

Lynn McKenzie, *Bark, Neigh Meow; Awaken to the Transformative Wisdom of Your Companion Animal to Activate Your Soul's Highest Calling*, Llewellyn Publications, 2021.

Kathleen Prasad, *Reiki for Dogs: Using Spiritual Energy to Heal and Vitalize Man's Best Friend*, Ulysses Press, 2021.

Martin J. Scott and Gael Mariani, *Crystal Healing for Animals*, Findhorn Press, 2002.

Diane Stein, *Natural Healing for Dogs and Cats*, Crossing Press, 1993.

Diane Stein, *The Natural Remedy Book for Dogs and Cats*, Crossing Press, 1994.

Online Sources and Websites

Daisy Foss, "7 Angels to Call Upon for Your Chakras", *Soul & Spirit*
www.soulandspiritmagazine.com/7-angels-call-upon-chakras/

Lynn McKenzie, Crystal Healing for Animals Home Study Program
www.lynnmckenzie.com/crystal-healing-for-animals/

Lynn McKenzie, Healing and Understanding Your Animal Companions through the Chakras™ Home Study Program
www.lynnmckenzie.com/healing-through-chakras/

Lynn McKenzie, The Chakra Balancing Method™ Home Study Program
www.lynnmckenzie.com/cbm/

Lynn McKenzie, *Animal Wellness* magazine author page
https://animalwellnessmagazine.com/author/lmckenzie/

Lynn McKenzie, *Equine Wellness* magazine author page
https://equinewellnessmagazine.com/author/lmckenzie/

Penelope Smith Animal Communication
www.AnimalTalk.net

INDEX

AUTHOR ACKNOWLEDGEMENTS

Thank you to all of my teachers, human and animal, with love and gratitude; especially to my beloved golden retriever, Jiggs, who came to me in the early 1990s to teach me, guide me and transform me. I had no idea what was in store for my life, and without your arrival I'd still be in a "normal" career and my current (and growing) body of work would not exist.

PICTURE CREDITS

Illustrations by Sian Summerhayes © Welbeck Non-Fiction Limited: 6, 8, 21, 29, 46, 50–1, 62, 70, 82, 88–9, 104, 114, 127, 128, 132.

Shutterstock: Alena Solonshchikova: 53, 55, 59, 63, 67, 71, 75, 79, 83, 87, 118, 120, 131, 135; An inspiration: 58, 66, 74, 78, 86; Anne Mathiasz: 52–8, 60–1, 63-6, 68–9, 71–4, 76–8, 80–1, 83–6; archivector: dog bullets throughout; graficriver_icons_logo: 5, 17, 111, 113, 119, pawprints throughout; HelloSSTK: 25, 49, 109, 138; jelisua88: 4–5, 41, 91–103; Nadzeya Shanchuk: 1, 18, 19, 24, 31, 35, 144; puaypuay: 12, 45, 92–102, 137; rame435: 107; UlMi: 19; yod 67: 18, 25, 49.

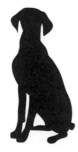